Contents

KU-762-799

Introduction

The purpose of this atlas is to provide the reader with an insight into the scope, the methods and the potential of the modern histopathology laboratory. It is not a textbook of pathology, of which many excellent examples are available. To the pathologist, most of the contents of this atlas will already be familiar. They will, however, inform the clinician of methods in current use as well as of their practicalities and snags. On the technical side, the medical laboratory scientific officer will be able to see the potential usefulness of techniques not already available to him or her, and may benefit from the presentation of artefacts and discussion on how to avoid them. The atlas should help the medical student to gain insight into the technical scope of modern histopathology. The layman, perhaps a hospital administrator, may learn what sort of work is done in a department of histopathology. We hope that readers of all kinds will enjoy the undoubted aesthetic qualities of tissues treated in many different ways which, in addition to providing important diagnostic information, often bring out their intrinsic beauty.

The atlas is divided into chapters, each dealing with a particular technique or aspect of laboratory work. The first chapter is concerned with that workhorse of histopathology, the paraffin section. On many occasions in the past (no doubt similar occasions will arise in the future), medical prophets have predicted the demise of the paraffin section. In the minds of these prophets, simple microscopy has been or will be replaced by electron microscopy, enzyme histochemistry, morphometry (the precise measurement and analysis of tissue components) or one of a number of other ways of handling or looking at tissues. Each of these has its place, but, strangely, the paraffin section remains. The situation is perhaps analogous to the survival, in an electronic age, of the simple stethoscope. Both have proved themselves over many years.

The next chapter deals with frozen sections, used both for rapid diagnosis and for techniques which require fresh, unembedded tissue.

Clinical Tests

Histopathology

P.J. Scheuer, D.Sc.(Med), M.D., F.R.C.Path.
B.T. Chalk, F.I.M.L.S.

Department of Histopathology
Royal Free Hospital and School of Medicine
London

Wolfe Medical Publications Ltd.

Copyright © P.J. Scheuer, B.T. Chalk 1986
Published by Wolfe Medical Publications Ltd 1986
Printed by Royal Smeets Offset B.V. The Netherlands
ISBN 0 7234 0885 8

General Editor, Wolfe Tests Series
D. Geraint James MA, MD (Cantab.), FRCP (London)

This book is one of the titles in the series of Wolfe Medical Atlases, a series which brings together probably the world's largest systematic published collection of diagnostic colour photographs.
   For a full list of Atlases in the series, plus forthcoming titles and details of our surgical, dental and veterinary Atlases, please write to Wolfe Medical Publications Ltd, Wolfe House, 3 Conway Street, London WIP 6HE.

The third chapter is on immunocytochemistry, the most rapidly growing technical area in histopathology. Basic immunocytochemical methods are now available in many laboratories, and not only in major centres. They provide an invaluable tool both in service work and in research. Next follows a chapter on specific histochemical methods for the identification of chemical substances in tissue; some of these were also included in the chapter on paraffin embedded tissue. Then follows a discussion of resin embedding for light microscopy, and a brief overview of present-day electron microscopy. Next, other forms of microscopy such as fluorescence and polarisation microscopy are discussed. Lastly, details are given of the methods illustrated. Except for brief reference in earlier chapters, the large and important topic of cytology has not been covered in the present volume.

The authors express the hope that the atlas will give instruction and enjoyment to its readers.

P.J. Scheuer
B.T. Chalk   London 1986

Acknowledgements

The authors wish to acknowledge the expert and generous help received throughout the preparation of this atlas by the staff of the Department of Histopathology at the Royal Free Hospital. Immunocytochemical methods were for the most part performed by Mrs. Alison West. Miss Jackie Lewin of the Electron Microscopy Unit provided electron micrographs. Mr. Paul Bates took the majority of the photographs of equipment and procedures. The manuscript was expertly typed by Miss Mary L. Mathias.

1 Paraffin sections

In this chapter we illustrate the procedures used for obtaining paraffin sections, and the results. A selection of commonly used stains is shown; others are included in Chapter 4. Illustrations of artefacts emphasise how these may interfere with accurate diagnosis.

The purpose of paraffin embedding is to provide a rigid support for optimally preserved tissues, enabling thin sections of high quality to be cut. Fresh tissue is first fixed to denature proteins, prevent autolysis and preserve as much structure as possible with minimum distortion and shrinkage. It is then dehydrated in a series of alcohols, cleared in an organic solvent and impregnated with molten wax or wax substitute. These procedures were first carried out by hand. In the last few decades processing machines have been developed, allowing automatic transfer of tissues from one reagent to another. Such machines now offer easy control over timing and temperature, so that each type of tissue is dealt with in the most appropriate way. The procedures have been made safer for laboratory workers by the development of enclosed apparatus which does not allow volatile reagents to escape into the atmosphere of the laboratory. After the tissue is embedded in a wax block it is cut on a microtome, usually to a thickness of between 2 and 6 μm. Sections are floated onto glass slides, deparaffinised, rehydrated, stained and mounted. Staining machines are available for applying routine stains such as haematoxylin and eosin to large numbers of sections. Finally, careful and accurate labelling reduces the possibility of error. The paraffin section remains the backbone of histological diagnosis in most laboratories. Accurate diagnosis by the pathologist often depends on the provision of paraffin sections of high quality.

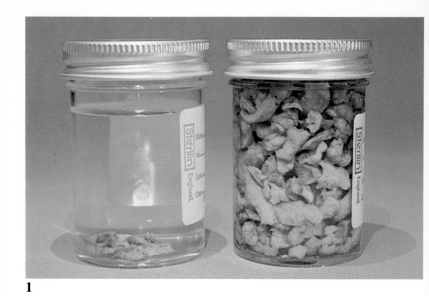

1

1   Fixing of the specimen On the left, the tissue has been placed in a suitable amount of fixative, many times the volume of the specimen itself. On the right, tissue has been crammed into the container. The amount of fixative in the latter is necessarily small in relation to the volume of the tissue, and fixation is likely to be poor.

2   Tissue examination and selection of blocks The pathologist is seen examining a surgical specimen. The macroscopic findings are noted, and pieces of tissue selected for paraffin processing. These tissue blocks should not measure more than approximately $2.5 \times 2.0 \times 0.4$ cm for optimum results.

3   Processing cassettes These are used to carry the tissue blocks through the various stages of the paraffin process. Each cassette is labelled with the specimen number, and the specimen is secured with a clip-on lid. The various colours can be used to code different types of specimens, e.g. surgical specimens, post mortem material and research material.

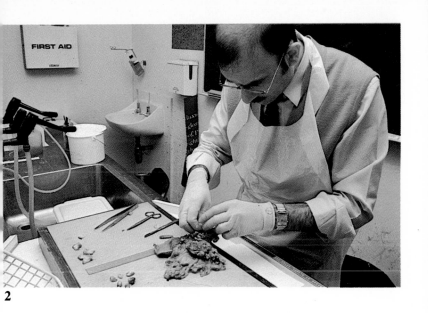

2

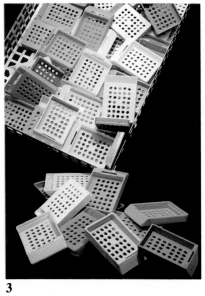

3

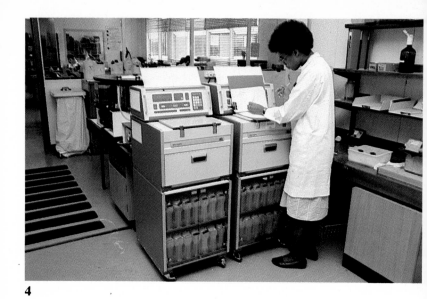

4

4   Tissue processing machine The equipment shown is totally enclosed, with a number of built-in safety features. This helps to keep the working environment free of fumes.

5   Paraffin embedding A modern paraffin embedding system is shown, with wax dispenser, hot plate and cooling stage. The latter enables paraffin blocks to be released quickly from the embedding moulds.

6   Section cutting Paraffin sections are being cut on a base sledge microtome, using a disposable knife blade. The thickness of the section can be varied at will. A thickness of 3 μm is common.

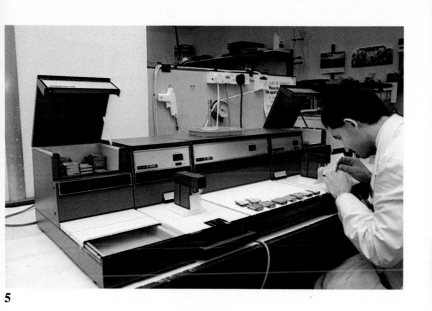

5

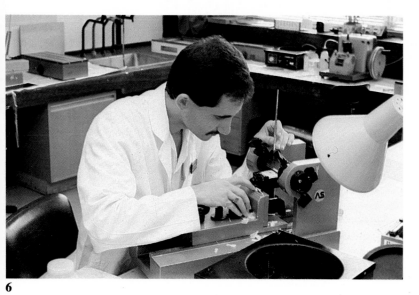

6

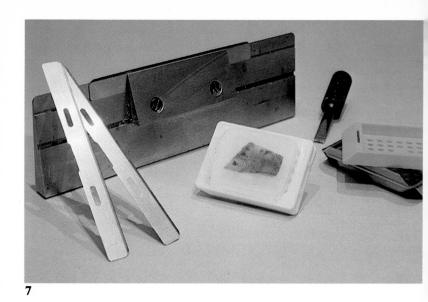

7

7   **Paraffin block and disposable knife** Disposable knives are shown together with a blade holder and screwdriver for fixing the blade. A cassette and lid are also seen.

8   **Section staining** Here a linear staining machine is being used for staining sections with haematoxylin and eosin. The glass slides are fixed to a slowly-moving chain drive, which allows them to pass through the different solutions. The number of troughs of each solution determines the length of exposure.

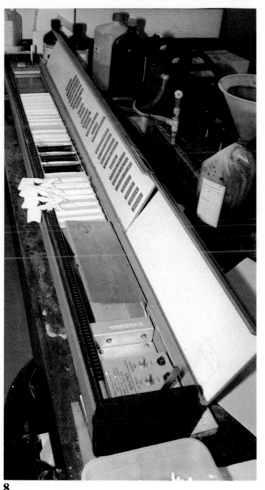

8

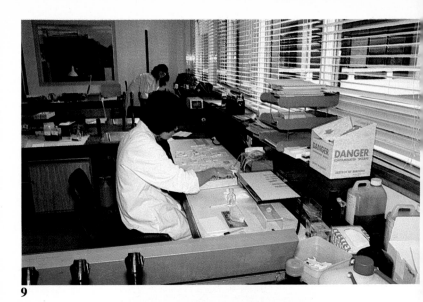

9

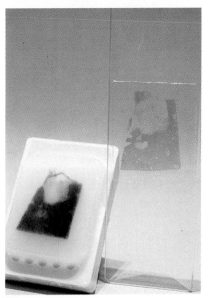

10

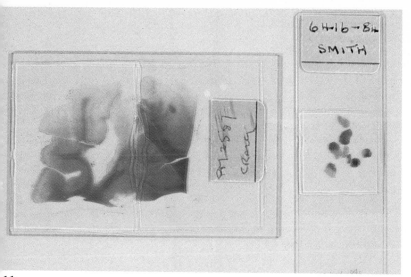

11

9 Mounting and labelling Good mounting is a skilled procedure. Accurate labelling is important to avoid possible errors (see **11**).

10 Paraffin block and section The section has been taken from the block, and is seen mounted but before labelling.

11 Good and bad mounting and labelling On the left is an example of an unevenly stained section which has also been poorly mounted using two separate cover glasses. The label is unclear. To the right is an example of a properly mounted and labelled slide.

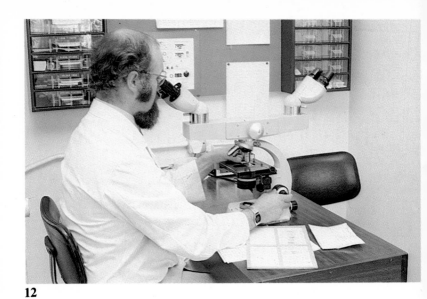

12

12 Quality control Here the finished section is being examined by an experienced technician under the microscope. Sections are checked for faults in cutting, staining, mounting and labelling.

13 Paraffin section: haematoxylin and eosin This example is from part of a benign breast lump, showing a variety of changes including apocrine metaplasia and epithelial proliferation. Fixation is good, and details are clear. No artefacts are seen.

14 Cautery artefact This sample of prostrate was removed by the surgeon with a cautery. The effects of coagulation are seen at the edge of the material. The staining is accentuated, and structure has been distorted.

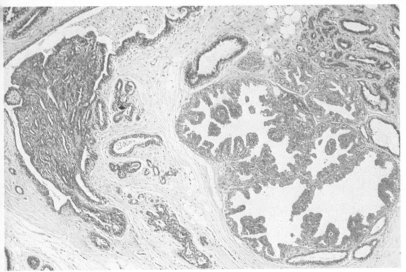

13

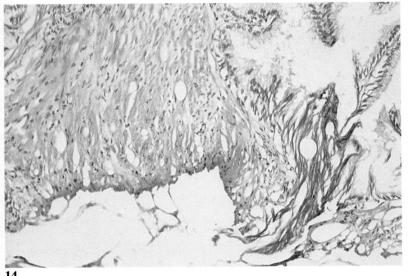

14

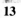

17

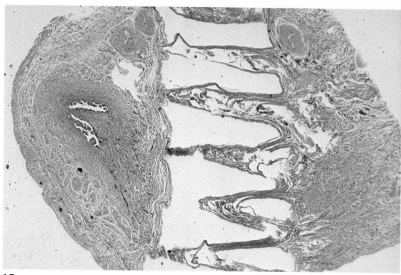

15

15 Forceps artefact The tissue has been roughly grasped with rat tooth forceps giving rise to the pattern of holes in the middle of the specimen. This has largely obliterated tissue structure, and has made diagnosis extremely difficult.

16 Freezing artefact This specimen of skin was frozen in error, before adequate fixation. The cells of the epidermis, which occupies much of the picture, appear vacuolated.

17 Iron artefact The tissue was transfixed with a pin. Iron has leached out of the pin into the adjacent tissue, and has given rise to artefactual positive staining with Perls' method for iron.

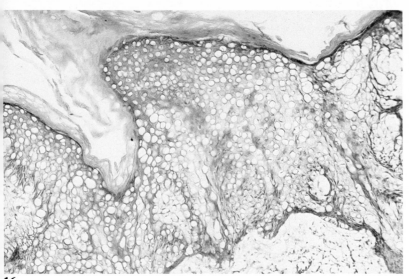

16

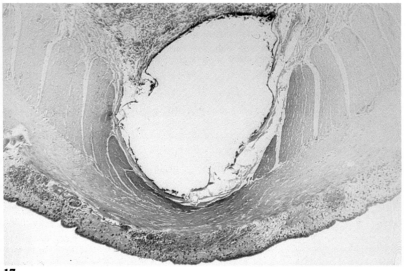

17

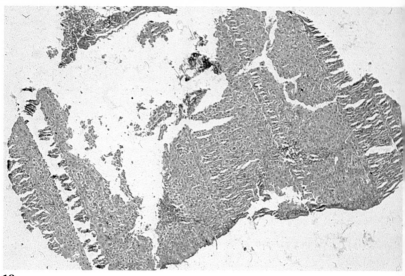

18

18 Sectioning artefact Here the fault lies in the cutting of the section. Linear parallel marks are due to imperfections in the microtome knife. Much of the tissue has been torn away. Diagnosis is virtually impossible in this liver biopsy.

19 Section mounting artefact The tissue has been roughly handled during transfer to a glass slide. Tears have developed, and there are folds of tissue obscuring much of the specimen.

20 Staining artefact Several irregular clumps of purple stain are seen lying on top of the otherwise well processed connective tissue.

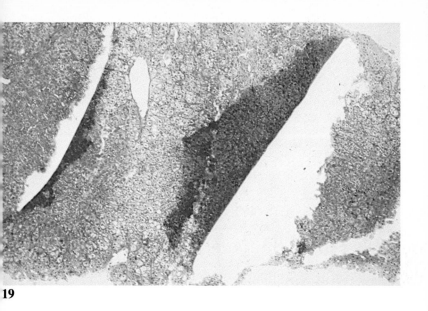

19

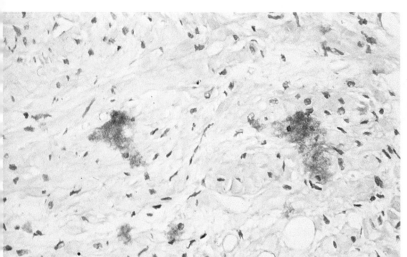

20

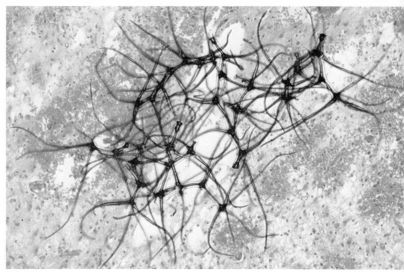

21

21 Mounting artefact The brown filaments represent pollens, introduced during the application of the cover slip. These pollens were present in the mounting medium.

22 Trichrome stain This is an example of the chromotrope aniline blue stain (CAB), applied to a liver biopsy. Preservation, sectioning, staining and mounting are satisfactory, and no artefacts are seen. Collagen fibres are stained blue, hepatocyte cytoplasm and nuclei purple, and erythrocytes bright red. There is perivenular fibrosis, the result of a healed lesion of alcoholic hepatitis.

23 Reticulin fibres A section of liver biopsy has been processed by Gordon and Sweets' silver method for reticulin fibres. These outline the hepatic sinusoids as well as the terminal hepatic venule (centrilobular vein) in the centre of the picture.

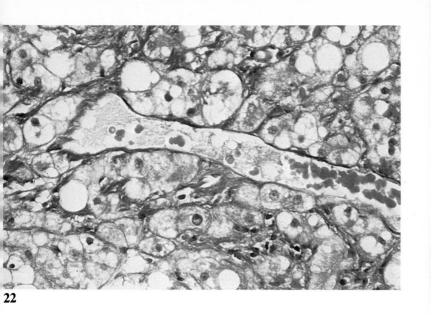

22

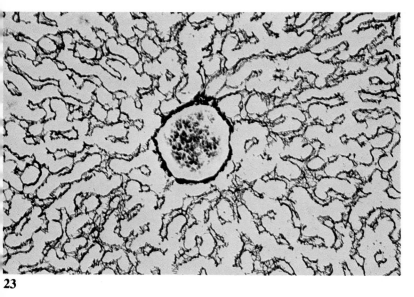

23

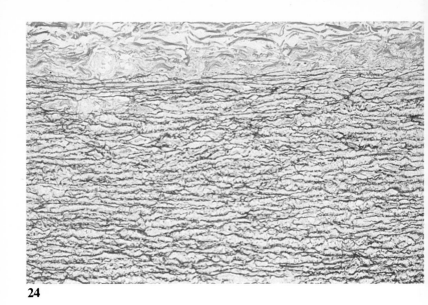

24

24 Elastic fibres Part of the wall of the aorta, showing approximately parallel laminae of elastic fibres, stained by the Miller-van Gieson method. Elastic fibres are dark brown, collagen fibres red.

25 Glycogen In this liver biopsy, glycogen has been stained by the periodic acid-Schiff (PAS) method and is seen as purple granular material within the cytoplasm of liver cells. Scanty fat vacuoles are also present. The glycogen is variable in amount because of partial solution in the aqueous reagents used in processing of the tissue and section.

26 Muscle striations The striations in fibres of voluntary muscle have been stained with phosphotungstic acid haematoxylin. Muscle fibres are purple, while collagen is stained red.

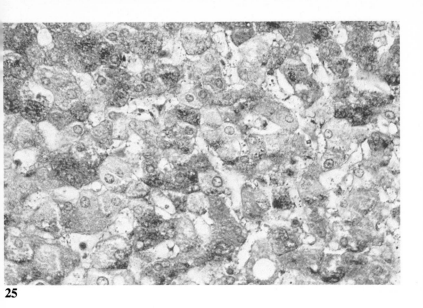

25

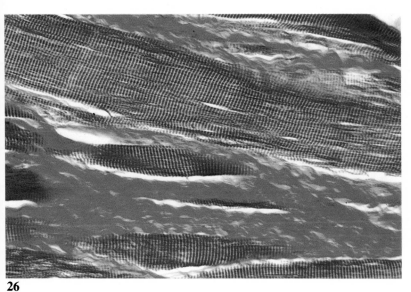

26

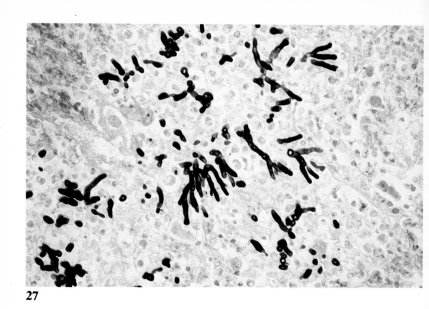

27

27 Grocott's method for fungi Hyphae of *Aspergillus* appear black in this silver method applied to a section of lung.

28 Ziehl-Neelsen stain for tubercle bacilli Many acid- and alcohol-fast bacilli, stained red, are seen in this section of lung. Compare with **80** (page 68).

29 Wade-Fite method for *M. leprae* Many leprosy bacilli are seen in the tissue in this example of the lepromatous form of leprosy. Their appearance is similar to but not identical with that of the organism of tuberculosis (**28**).

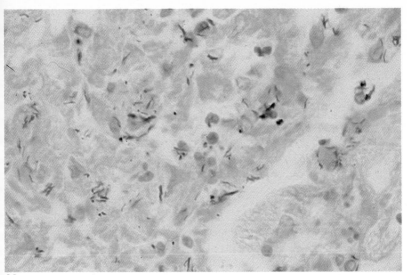

28

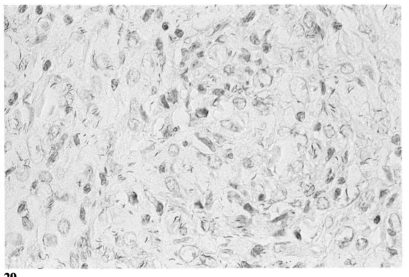

29

2   Frozen sections

Frozen sections are used when paraffin sections are unsuitable, either because of the need for a rapid result or because tissue components such as lipids or antigens are removed or destroyed during the embedding process. While frozen sections are generally inferior to paraffin sections and are less easily preserved, they can be produced to a high standard with modern equipment. Best results are obtained with solid tissues.

The unfixed tissue is rapidly frozen, allowing thin sections to be cut on a cryostat, which is essentially a microtome with remote controls, housed in a freezing cabinet. Sections can be produced and stained in the course of a few minutes, whereas paraffin sections take some hours at best. Frozen sections are therefore suitable for rapid diagnosis of lesions sampled or excised by the surgeon during an operation, when a therapeutic decision needs to be made. Other methods for rapid diagnosis, the imprint and the smear, are also illustrated in this chapter. Frozen sections are widely used in immunocytochemistry, because of good preservation of tissue antigens. Other uses of frozen sections include the demonstration of enzymes, lipids and certain cellular structures of the nervous system.

30   Cryostat This refrigerated microtome is used for cutting frozen sections from fresh, unfixed tissue. The temperature can be varied from −10°C to −30°C.

31   Detail of cryostat This shows the microtome within the cabinet, with its knife and anti-roll plate. The latter keeps the sections flat. All controls are externally placed, and the sections can be cut at approximately 5 μm. They are then picked up onto clean glass slides and stained by appropriate methods.

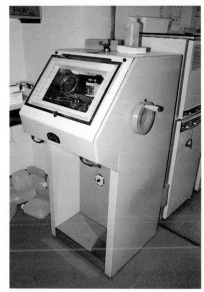

30

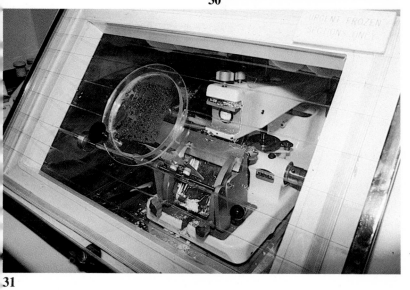

31

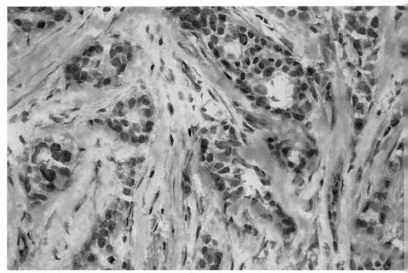

32

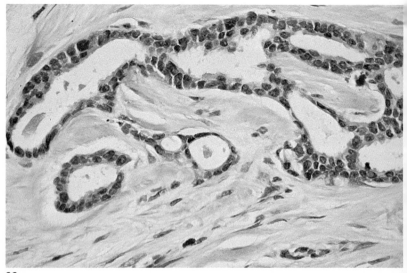

33

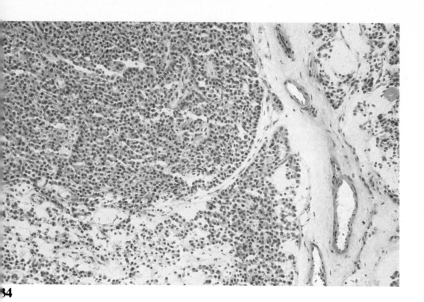

34

32   Frozen section of breast A high power view of part of an invasive carcinoma of breast as seen in a cryostat section stained with haematoxylin and eosin. The tumour is easily recognised and the quality of the section is sufficient for rapid diagnosis.

33   Paraffin section of breast This section is from the same tumour seen in **32**. Following frozen sectioning, other tissue from the same tumour was fixed and embedded in paraffin. The overall appearances are similar, but detail is better preserved than in the cryostat section.

34   Frozen section of parathyroid A common reason for frozen section request is the identification of tissue at parathyroidectomy. Shown here is a frozen section which includes nodular hyperplastic parathyroid tissue.

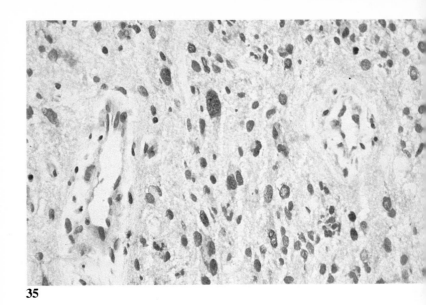

35

35 Frozen section of brain Frozen sections are widely used in neurosurgery to establish whether material consists of tumour or not. This cryostat section shows an astrocytoma composed of large cells with hyperchromatic nuclei. Two blood vessels with prominent lining cells are also seen.

36 Bad frozen section of brain Here poor sectioning technique has produced distorted strips of tissue instead of an even, coherent section. The tissue is still recognisable as an astrocytoma, but in other instances diagnosis might be made difficult or impossible by the poor quality of a section. Compare with **35**.

37 Brain smear This has been prepared by smearing material obtained for rapid diagnosis on a glass slide. The smear was stained with haematoxylin and eosin. The large cells are part of a tumour of the type seen in **35** and **36**.

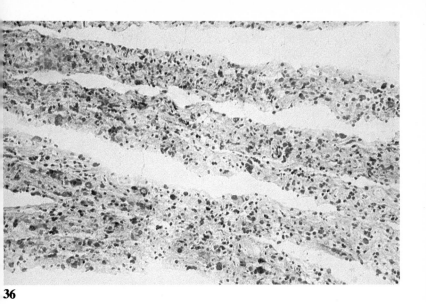

36

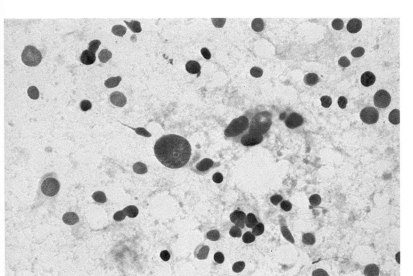

37

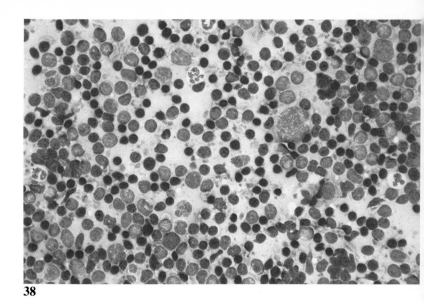

38

38 Imprint of lymph node This is another method for rapid diagnosis. The cut surface of a lymph node has been briefly applied to a glass slide, and the surface cells have adhered to the glass. The morphology of the cells is well preserved. A variety of lymphoid cells and segmented leucocytes can be identified in this preparation, together with large cells of Hodgkin's disease. The section has been stained with haematoxylin and eosin.

39 Cajal's gold chloride method Here a frozen section has been used for a stain which cannot be satisfactorily performed on paraffin embedded material. The high power view shows darkly stained astrocytes with many long processes.

40 Frozen section stained for fat Part of the adrenal cortex is seen, stained for fat with oil red O. Many bright red fat globules are seen in the epithelial cells. This type of stain has to be performed on frozen sections because fat is dissolved during the processing of material for paraffin embedding.

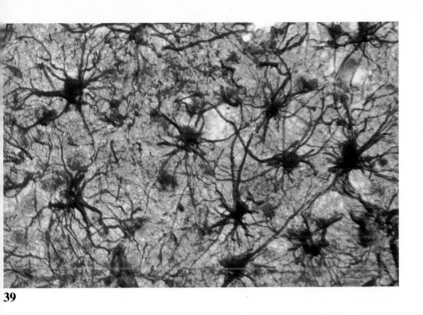

39

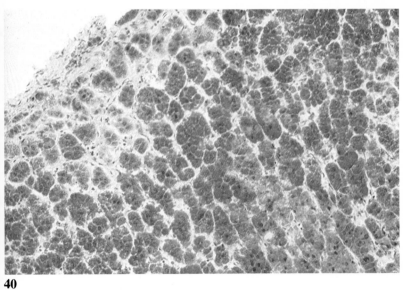

40

3 Immunocytochemistry

Immunocytochemical methods now play an important part in many histopathology laboratories. Antigens are identified in frozen or paraffin sections by means of specific polyclonal or monoclonal antibodies. These are either labelled directly with a marker such as a fluorescent dye, or a further layer or layers are added to complete the reaction. As will be seen from the illustrations, a wide range of substances can be displayed. They include tissue enzymes, which can thus be shown either by immunocytochemistry by virtue of their antigenic properties, or by a histochemical technique such as the ones discussed in the next chapter.

Immunocytochemistry requires strict attention to both negative and positive controls, in order to avoid misleading results. For further details the reader is referred to a number of recent publications, given in the section on Further reading (page 126).

41 Renal glomerulus: immunofluorescence The section has been stained for IgG, using an antibody conjugated with a fluorescent dye (FITC). The green fluorescence indicates the sites of IgG deposition.

42 Double fluorescent staining A group of B lymphocytes has been stained for kappa and lambda light chains, using two different fluorescent dyes. Kappa chains are stained green, and lambda chains orange. The nuclei are seen as dark, round, unstained areas in each cell.

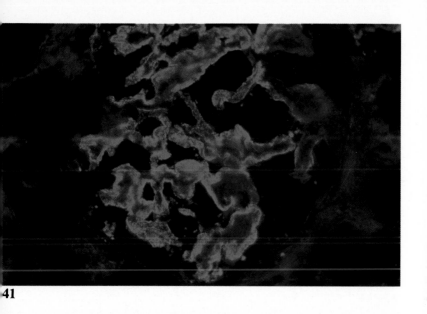

41

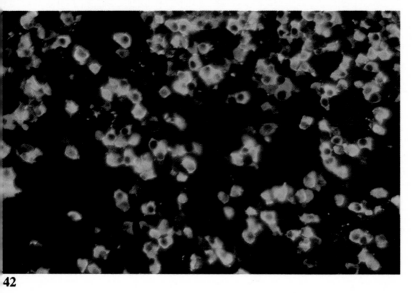

42

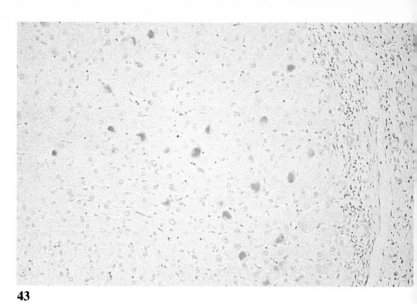

43

44

38

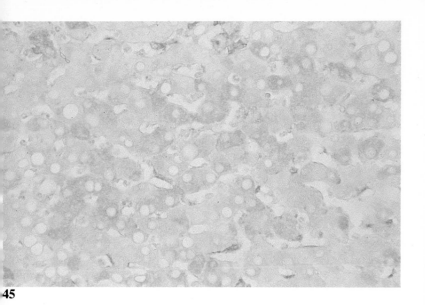

45

43   Immunoperoxidase method for hepatitis B surface antigen Part of a cirrhotic nodule is seen, in which scattered hepatocytes are stained brown. A specific antibody to hepatitis B surface antigen was used.

44   Negative control section Adjacent section to that seen in **43**, showing the negative control in which the specific antiserum was omitted. The background is totally devoid of brown stain.

45   Artefactual background staining The antibody used here was one against β_2-microglobulin, conjugated with peroxidase. Many hepatocytes in this liver have brown cytoplasm, while the nuclei have remained unstained. Elongated sinusoidal cells are also positive. The intracytoplasmic staining of hepatocytes, which is seen particularly at the edge of operative wedge biopsies, is probably an artefact. Contrast with the clean background of **44**.

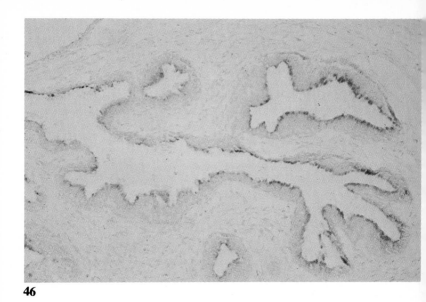

46

46 Prostatic acid phosphatase In this section the enzyme has been demonstrated by an immunological method using a red dye, 3-amino-9-ethylcarbazole, as a marker. The enzyme is seen in the cytoplasm of prostatic epithelial cells lining the glands.

4 Histochemical techniques

Histochemical methods not based on immunological reactions are used to identify specific chemical substances in tissues. These may be enzymes (**47, 48**), metals (**49, 50**) or other substances. Histochemistry offers a functional, biochemical approach to histological diagnosis and permits more accurate identification than is possible in conventional haematoxylin and eosin sections. It should be noted, however, that even routine stains are based on histochemical reactions (see Chapter 1). Thus, for example, haematoxylin and eosin broadly distinguishes acidic substances such as nucleic acids and mucins, stained blue, from basic substances which stain with the acid eosin.

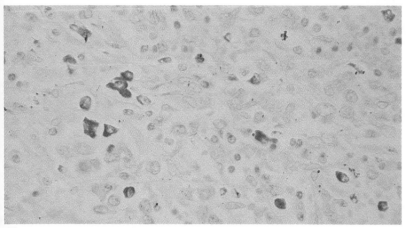

47

47 Histochemical method for acid phosphatase Macrophages containing abundant acid phosphatase in their cytoplasm have been stained red in this frozen section of tonsil. In contrast to **46**, phosphatase has here been demonstrated by means of a purely histochemical technique not involving an immunological reaction. The section has been treated with a phosphate substrate and a buffer. Following the action of enzyme in the cytoplasm of the cells, a red insoluble azo dye was deposited.

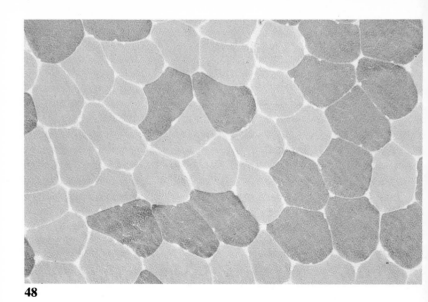

48

48 ATPase in muscle A histochemical method has been used to demonstrate enzyme activity in type 2 fibres.

49 Perls' stain for iron Part of a liver biopsy showing abundant deposits of iron, stained blue with the Prussian blue method, in hepatocytes.

50 Rhodanine stain for copper A liver biopsy with abundant deposits of copper in the form of red-stained granules in hepatocytes.

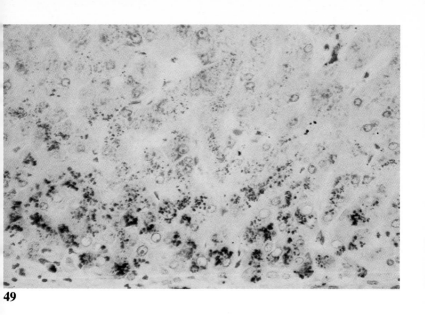

49

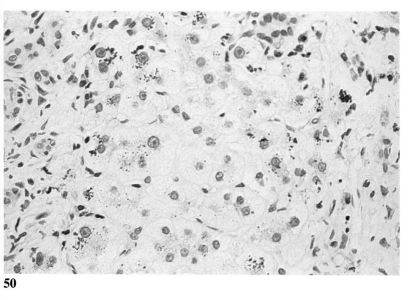

50

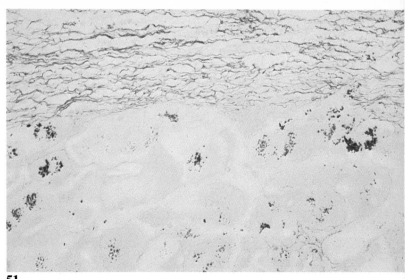

51

51 Orcein stain for copper-associated protein and elastic fibres A protein closely associated with copper (50) has been demonstrated by the orcein method. The protein is seen as dark granules in hepatocytes adjacent to connective tissue (top). Elastic fibres in the latter are stained. The orcein method is also used for the demonstration of hepatitis B surface antigen.

52 Alcian blue-PAS stain for mucins This composite method is used for the demonstration of both neutral and acid mucins. The former are stained by the PAS method after amylase (diastase) digestion (see also **25**) while acid mucins are stained blue with alcian blue. In this example, both types of mucin are seen in a salivary gland.

53 Masson Fontana method for melanin The illustration shows melanocytes in the epidermis, identified by their dense black cytoplasm. The nuclei have remained unstained. The method is often used in the diagnosis of malignant melanoma.

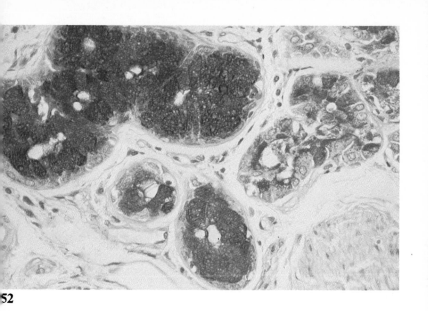

52

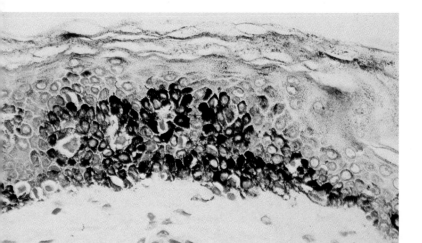

53

45

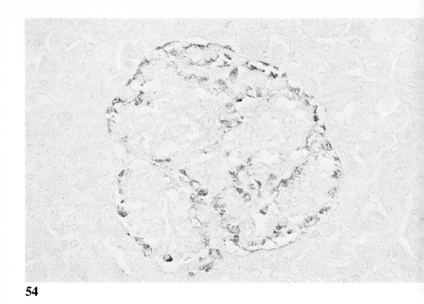

54

54 Neurosecretory granules in a pancreatic islet The Grimelius silver method has been used to demonstrate cells containing neurosecretory granules in a normal pancreatic islet. The method is also used to identify similar granules in tumours of the carcinoid or APUD-cell type.

55 Linder method for neurosecretory granules A different silver method from the one used in **54** has here been applied to a carcinoid tumour of the appendix. Black granules are seen in many of the tumour cells, and establish the nature of the lesion. Further confirmation could be obtained by electron microscopy (**70**).

56 Tripp-MacKay method for calcified bone and osteoid This silver method is used for the demonstration of osteoid, especially in the diagnosis of osteomalacia in which excess osteoid is formed. Decalcification, which is necessary for the cutting of paraffin sections, makes it difficult to distinguish between calcified and uncalcified bone. A silver solution is therefore used before embedding of the tissue, to show the calcified areas. These are black in the picture, whereas uncalcified osteoid is stained red.

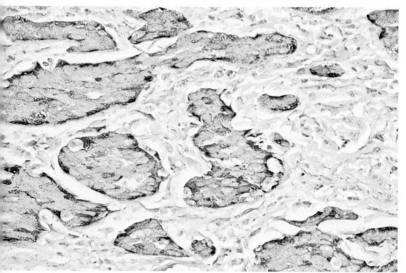

55

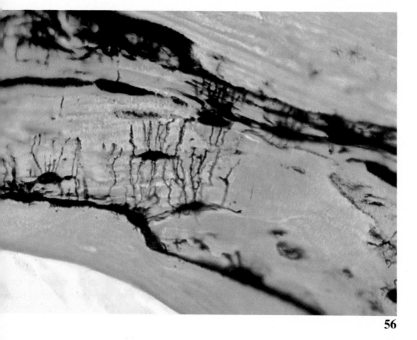

56

5 Resin sections: light microscopy

Tissues may be embedded in plastic resins instead of paraffin. Such resins are in some instances the same as those used for electron microscopy, but special materials have also been developed for light microscopy. The resin-embedded sections can be cut on special microtomes with great accuracy to produce sections 1 or 2 μm thick. This is particularly helpful when accurate cytological detail is required. The range of stains which can be carried out is usually somewhat more restricted than for paraffin sections, but with some resins most routine procedures are possible, and even immunohistochemical techniques can be used (as shown in **61**).

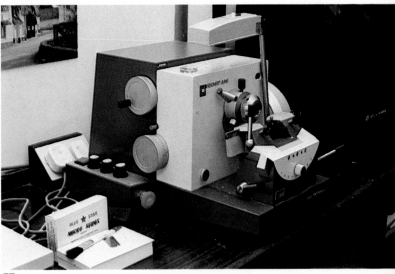

57

57 Microtome for resin sections This specially designed, motor-driven microtome is used to cut resin-embedded blocks for light microscopy. Sections are cut at 1 – 2μm, placed on glass slides, stained and mounted.

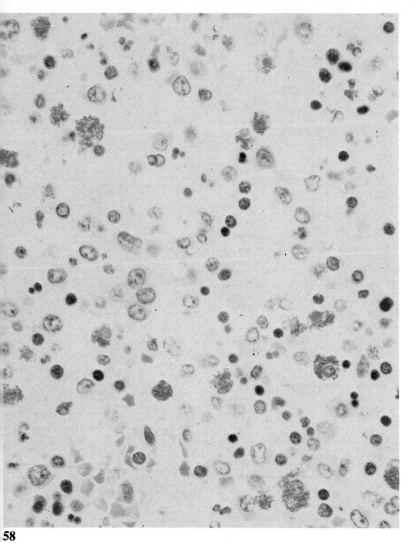

58

58 **Resin section of bone marrow** In this high power view, individual marrow cells are clearly shown, with good detail of nuclear structure and cytoplasmic granules. Eosinophil precursors are easily identified by their content of bright red granules. Detail is much better preserved than in paraffin sections. The stain is haematoxylin and eosin.

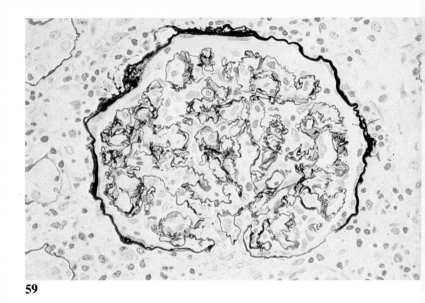

59

59   Resin section of kidney The basement membranes of a glomerulus appear black by the hexamine (methenamine) silver method. This glomerulus is histologically within normal limits. The good preservation of detail allows epithelial, endothelial and mesangial cells to be identified and separately assessed.

60   Amylase PAS stain of resin section In the example of liver in a patient with α_1-antitrypsin deficiency, many of the hepatocytes contain purple-stained globules of different sizes. The resin used in this instance was of a water soluble type.

61   Immunoperoxidase stain on resin section The specimen is the one shown in **60**. The section has been stained by the immunoperoxidase method, using an antibody against α_1- antitrypsin. The globules, corresponding to the ones shown in **60**, are clearly seen.

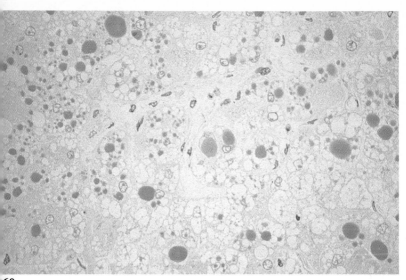

60

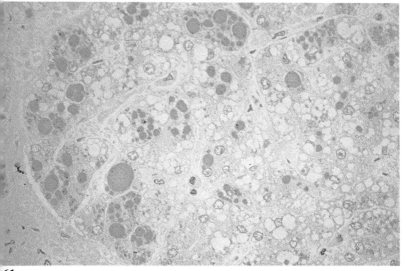

61

6   Resin sections: electron microscopy

The development of electron microscopy has greatly extended the scope of the morphological sciences, and has played its part in the recent explosion of understanding of the mammalian cell. Tissues can be viewed in the transmission mode, in which the light beam of the conventional microscope is replaced by a beam of electrons generated at high voltage at the top of a long column (67). Alternatively, surfaces can be viewed in a scanning electron microscope (73) after suitable preparation. X-ray microanalysis (73) makes it possible to identify individual elements in the tissue.

Electron microscopy is a powerful tool in biological and other research, but is also used for diagnosis. In human pathology it has a particular place in the identification of tumours (70) and abnormal storage products (69).

Specimens for transmission electron microscopy need to be fixed very rapidly to avoid artefacts. Processing can be automated, as in the case of paraffin embedding. The final product is a hard resin block (65, 66) containing a minute fragment of tissue, usually less than 1 mm across. The block is cut on a special microtome, using a glass or diamond knife, and put on a metal grid which is then inserted into the microscope.

62   Processing machine for electron microscopy This modern tissue processor allows the minute specimens used in electron microscopy to be processed automatically. Reagents can be used in very small, accurately measured quantities and the exact programme is controlled by a microcomputer. The end result of the process is a resin block containing the specimen (see 65 and 66).

63   Ultramicrotome This is used for cutting ultra-thin sections from resin-embedded tissue for examination in a transmission electron microscope, in which the electron beam passes through the specimen. Sections are cut with a diamond or glass knife to a thickness of 30–80 nm. The binocular attachment enables the very small specimen to be accurately seen and sectioned.

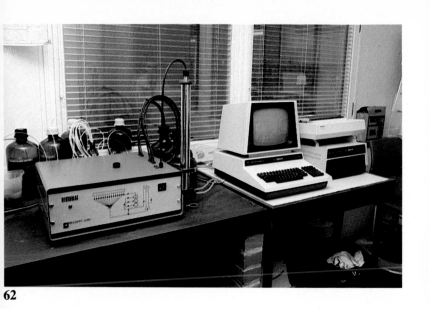

62

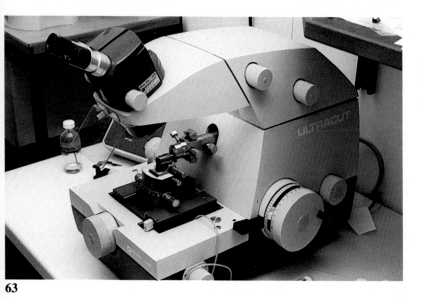

63

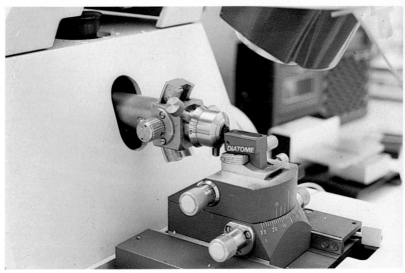

64

64   Ultramicrotome Here the sectioning part of the ultramicrotome is seen in close-up. Sections are floated onto ethanol or acetone contained in the blue trough, and picked up on a copper grid.

65   Blocks, knives and grids Here resin blocks containing minute amounts of tissue are seen, together with glass knives and the copper grids on which sections are placed. The scale is shown by the drawing pins. The grids are put in the electron beam of the transmission microscope by means of a specimen holder.

66   Blocks for electron and light microscopy A paraffin block for light microscopy (right) and resin-embedded tissue for electron microscopy (left). The pencil tip gives an indication of size.

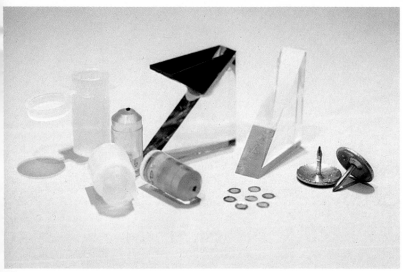

65

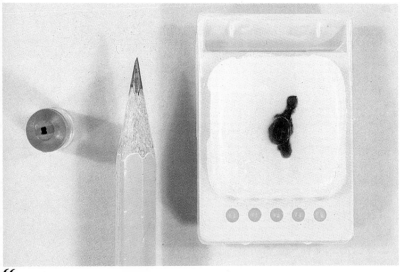

66

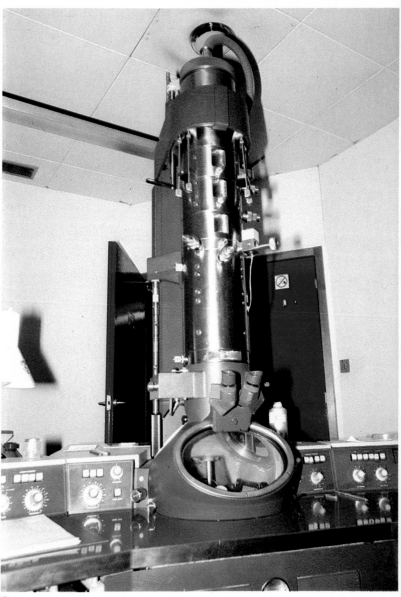

67

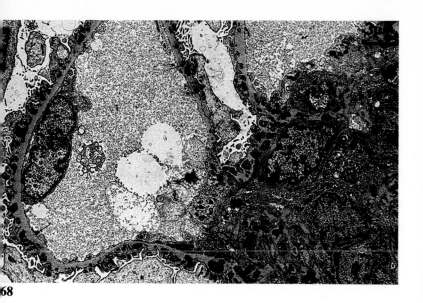

68

67   Transmission electron microscope The electron beam passes through the tall column, within which the specimen is placed. At the top of the column is the electron gun, connected to a high voltage cable. The viewing chamber and controls are seen below.

68   Renal glomerulus by transmission electron microscopy The lumen (1) contains flocculent material. An endothelial cell (2) is seen closely applied to the basement membrane (arrow). Mesangial tissue is shown on the right.

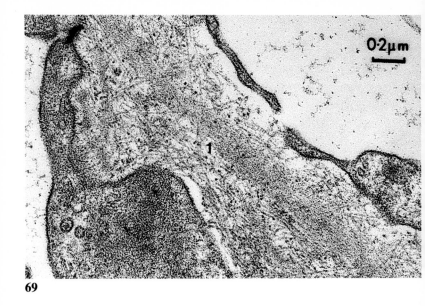

69

69 Amyloid in glomerular basement membrane by transmission electron microscopy The basement membrane has been largely replaced by amyloid, composed of characteristic fibrils (1). Parts of endothelial and epithelial cells are seen on either side.

70 Carcinoid tumour: transmission electron microscopy Parts of several tumour cells are seen, containing abundant electron dense neurosecretory granules (arrow). The nuclei (1) have irregular outlines.

71 Adenovirus: transmission electron microscopy Virus particles (arrows) have been demonstrated by means of negative staining. Note the crystalline structure of the virus particles.

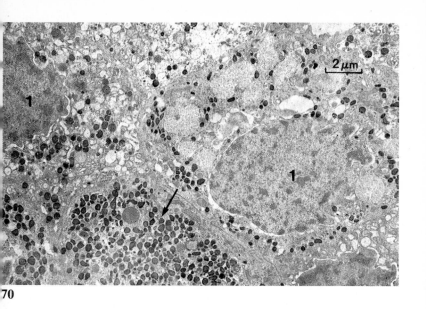

70

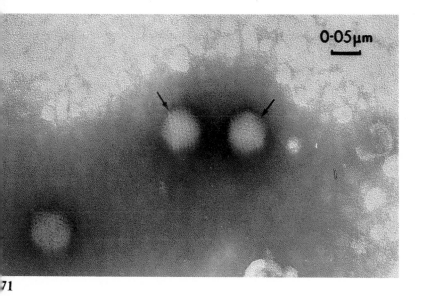

71

59

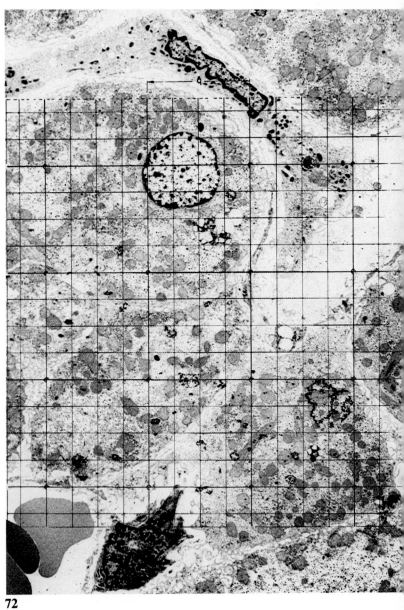

72

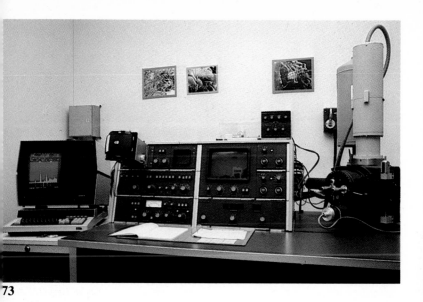

73

72 Morphometry A variety of morphometric techniques can be applied to tissues both at light- and electron-microscopic level. Here a grid has been superimposed on an electron micrograph of human liver. The number of grid intersections falling on any particular structure (e.g. nucleus, mitochondria, sinusoidal lumen) gives an indication of the relative volumes of these structures in the tissue, provided that the sample is of adequate size.

73 Scanning electron microscope and X-ray microanalysis The column is seen to the right of the figure, and the specimen is inserted into the black chamber below the column. The screen (centre) is for viewing the image, and to the left there is part of the X-ray microanalysis equipment. The orange spikes on the screen represent concentrations of elements in the tissue under examination.

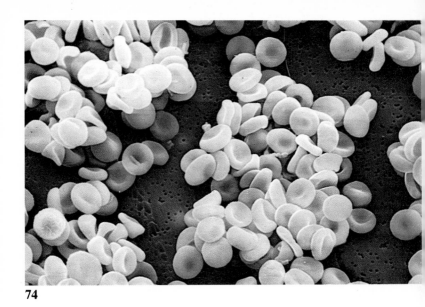

74

74 **Human red blood cells viewed by scanning electron microscopy** The biconcave shape of the cells is clearly seen.

7   Special techniques of microscopy

This section deals with techniques in light microscopy other than those already illustrated. Fluorescence microscopy has an important place in the laboratory because of its widespread use in immunocytochemistry, where fluorescent markers are used. Fluorescent dyes are also used for the identification of a variety of chemical substances including amyloid (79). Fluorescent staining for tubercle bacilli enables small numbers to be identified at a relatively low magnification (80). Polarising microscopy is a standard procedure for the histopathologist, and as far as possible every pathologist should have a polariser fitted to his or her microscope. This is not only useful for the identification of amyloid after staining with Congo red and foreign substances such as suture material, but also for the assessment of normal tissue components such as collagen (75).

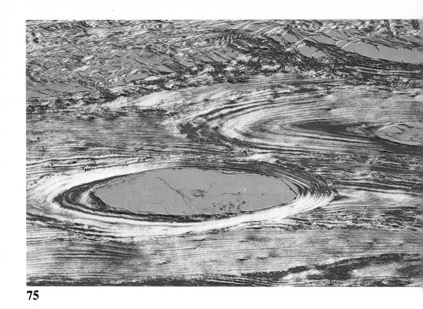

75

75 Bone by polarising microscopy The regular lines seen in this lamellar bone under polarised light represent layers of collagen in the organic matrix of the bone. Polarisation is used to distinguish between mature, lamellar bone and newly-formed, woven bone.

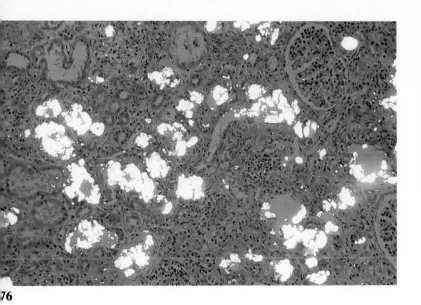

76

76   Oxalate crystals in kidney The crystalline structure of oxalates makes them brightly birefringent under polarised light, as seen in this specimen of human kidney.

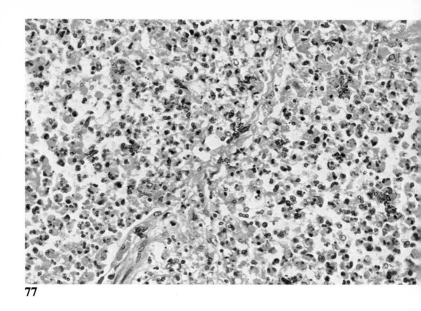

77

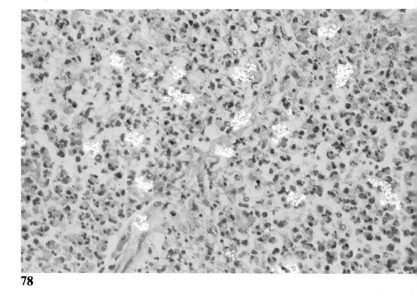

78

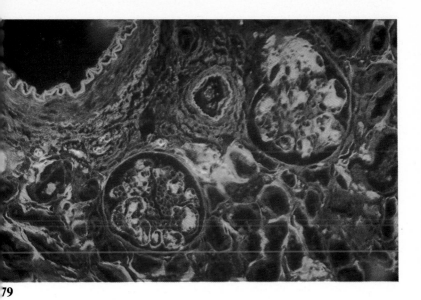

79

77　**Mercury pigment** In specimens fixed in solutions containing mercury salts, these should be removed before staining. Here the mercury salts have not been removed, and are seen as brown crystalline deposits.

78　**Mercury pigment, polarised light** The same field as 77 under polarised light, showing the bright birefringence of the mercury pigment. Polarisation is one of the methods which help to distinguish different pigments under the microscope.

79　**Amyloid stained with thioflavine T** Bright amyloid deposits are seen in glomeruli and around renal tubules.

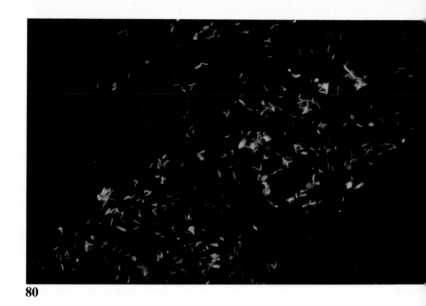

80

80 *M. tuberculosis* stained with auramine-rhodamine Tubercle bacilli give a bright golden fluorescence when stained with auramine-rhodamine. This enables even small numbers of the organisms to be detected at relatively low magnifications. The method is thus very useful when searching large areas of tissue. Compare with the same bacilli stained by the Ziehl-Neelsen method (**28**).

Staining methods

The staining and impregnating techniques which follow are those referred to in the illustrations in the first part of this book. The techniques are listed step by step and certain steps are given in an abbreviated form. The commonly used abbreviations are as follows:

1. 'Sections to water' (or alcohol)

As most staining solutions are either aqueous or alcoholic it is necessary to treat paraffin sections with a wax solvent (e.g. xylene). After treatment with xylene (which is not miscible with water) the sections are treated with descending grades of ethyl alcohol diluted with distilled water. The sections are then finally placed in water prior to carrying out the staining technique. Certain staining techniques use alcoholic solutions of dyes and it is therefore necessary to transfer the sections from absolute ethyl alcohol to these solutions. If sections are transferred from water to alcoholic solutions of dyes, precipitation of the dye can occur on the section.

The technique of taking sections to water is as follows:

(a) Warm paraffin sections until the wax just melts. Do not overheat the sections as this can interfere with some staining techniques.

(b) Remove the wax by treating the sections with xylene. This usually takes at least 5 minutes and it is advisable to change the dewaxing xylene two or three times during this period. Because of the hazardous nature of xylene this chemical should be used under an extraction hood. There are other wax solvents which are less toxic than xylene but experience has shown that these are not as satisfactory for dewaxing.

(c) Remove the xylene by treating the sections with absolute ethyl alcohol (or isopropyl alcohol). Treat the sections with 90 per cent alcohol and then with 70 per cent alcohol. The sections can now be transferred to water.

2. 'Washing with water'

Where necessary the techniques indicate the times for washing with either tap or distilled water. The term 'running tap water' means that the sections are placed in a tray or glass trough and tap water is gently run over the sections via tubing connected to the tap. Some staining techniques require washing in running tap water for at least 5 to 10 minutes in order to remove excess stains or chemicals from the section prior to the next step in the technique. The use of very large quantities of distilled water for washing sections is indicated in certain metallic impregnating techniques. Tap water, if used in these techniques, will cause precipitation of the metallic salts.

3. 'Staining at room temperature'

Room temperatures in the United Kingdom are usually between 18°C and 22°C. It is important to note that any decrease or increase in the stated temperatures will affect the staining times.

4. 'Dehydrate, clear and mount'

Once the staining technique has been completed the section must be permanently sealed under a thin cover glass. The mountant used can be either a synthetic or natural resinous medium. These mountants are not miscible with water or alcohol. In certain techniques, e.g. oil red O for lipids, alcohol or xylene must not be used as they will dissolve the lipid. In this method the sections are mounted from water using an aqueous mountant (e.g. Apathy's syrup).

The technique for mounting using a synthetic or natural resin is as follows:
(a) Dehydration is achieved by passing the sections through ascending grades of ethyl alcohol (70 per cent, 90 per cent) to absolute ethyl alcohol. This stage is critical as any trace of water in the section, if not removed, will show as a 'milky' film on the section when mounted.
(b) Clearing in xylene will remove the alcohol from the section. This usually requires two to three changes of xylene.
(c) Mounting of the section using a coverglass requires a certain amount of skill; in the hands of the inexperienced it can be messy. Drain the excess xylene from the section and place the section, face up, on the bench. Place a drop of mountant on the section, avoiding air bubbles in the drop of mountant. These bubbles will be difficult to remove once the coverglass has been placed on the section and may give rise, later, to retraction of the mountant. Gently lower the coverglass on to the section at an angle, allowing the mountant to spread across the section evenly without trapping air bubbles. Any excess mountant can be wiped away using tissue paper or a fluff-free cloth. Most synthetic mountants will harden sufficiently after 24 hours. The use of a 56°C oven will shorten the drying time.

5. 'Removal of mercury pigment'

Certain fixatives which contain mercuric chloride give rise to artefactual deposition of pigment in tissues. It is therefore necessary to remove this pigment by treating the section, prior to staining, with Lugol's iodine for 3 to 5 minutes. The section is washed in running tap water for 1 minute and then treated with 1 per cent aqueous sodium thiosulphate ('hypo') for 1 minute. After washing in running tap water for 1 minute the section is ready for staining.

6. 'Celloidinisation'

Some tissues when paraffin processed tend to be friable. This can give rise to the sections 'floating off' the glass slide when performing staining techniques. To overcome this problem, the sections can be coated with a film of a weak celloidin solution. This technique is often useful when carrying out methods which use ammoniacal solutions.

The technique is as follows:

(a) Carefully dewax sections with xylene in the usual way.
(b) Treat sections with absolute alcohol to remove xylene.
(c) Blot sections, almost dry, with best quality blotting paper.
(d) Dip the sections in a solution of 1 per cent celloidin in equal parts ether–alcohol.
(e) Air-dry the coated sections for about 20 seconds.
(f) Place sections in 70 per cent alcohol for 30 seconds.
(g) Wash sections in running tap water for 1 minute.

The sections are now ready for staining. The celloidin film can be removed, if required, after staining by placing the sections in acetone.

ALCIAN BLUE – PAS TECHNIQUE
(for acid and neutral mucins)

Reference: Mowry R.W. (1956) *Journal of Histochemistry and Cytochemistry* **4**, 407

Solutions

1 per cent alcian blue in 3 per cent aqueous acetic acid
1 per cent aqueous periodic acid
Schiff's reagent (see page 124)
Carazzi's haematoxylin (see page 116)
1 per cent hydrochloric acid in 70 per cent alcohol
2 per cent aqueous sodium bicarbonate

Technique

1   Take test section and control section to distilled water.
2   Stain with the alcian blue solution for 5 minutes.
3   Wash well in distilled water for 2 minutes.
4   Treat with 1 per cent periodic acid solution for 5 minutes.
5   Wash in several changes of distilled water for 2 minutes.
6   Treat with Schiff's reagent for 10 minutes.
7   Wash the sections in running tap water for 10 minutes (this will intensify the colour of the Schiff positive material).
8   Stain the nuclei with Carazzi's haematoxylin for 2 minutes.
9   Differentiate in acid alcohol for 1–2 seconds.
10 Wash well in tap water for two minutes.
11 'Blue' the sections in 2 per cent sodium bicarbonate.
12 Wash well in running tap water for 5 minutes.
13 Dehydrate, clear and mount.

Results

Acid mucins	blue
Neutral mucins	magenta
Mixtures of both	purple
Nuclei	pale blue

Notes

1 This technique is most useful in distinguishing between acid and neutral mucins.
2 The nuclear counterstain must be light as overstaining with haematoxylin can give rise to cytoplasmic staining, which will give confusing results with the alcian blue. Carazzi's haematoxylin is recommended for this technique.

ALKALINE DIAZO TECHNIQUE FOR ENTEROCHROMAFFIN CELLS

Reference: Gomori G. (1952) *Microscopic Histochemistry*, Chicago; Chicago University Press

Solutions

1 per cent aqueous fast red B (freshly prepared)
Saturated aqueous lithium carbonate
Carazzi's haematoxylin (see page 116)

Technique

1 Take test section and control section to distilled water.
2 Mix 5 parts fast red B solution (precooled to 4°C) with 2 parts saturated lithium carbonate (precooled to 4°C). Filter the solution into a Coplin jar.
3 Transfer sections to the filtered diazonium solution and leave for 1–4 minutes at 4°C.
4 Rinse sections in distilled water for 20 seconds.
5 Wash sections well in running tap water for 5 minutes.
6 Stain sections with Carazzi's haematoxylin for 2 minutes.
7 Wash well in running tap water for 2–3 minutes.
8 Dehydrate, clear and mount.

Results

Enterochromaffin cell granules	orange–red
Nuclei	blue
Background	yellow

Notes

1 Tissue freshly fixed in formalin gives best results.
2 This method rarely works on postmortem material.
3 Some batches of the diazonium salt may give poor results and all batches have a limited shelf life.

AURAMINE–RHODAMINE TECHNIQUE
(for tubercle and leprosy bacilli)

Reference: Silver A., Sonnenwirth A.C., Alex N. (1966) *Journal of Clinical Pathology* **19**, 583

Solutions

Auramine–rhodamine solution (see page 115)
0.5 per cent hydrochloric acid in 70 per cent alcohol (for tubercle bacilli)
0.5 per cent aqueous hydrochloric acid (for leprosy bacilli)
0.5 per cent aqueous potassium permanganate

Technique

1 Take the test section and control section to water.
2 Stain the sections in filtered auramine–rhodamine solution, preheated to 56°C, for 10 minutes.
3 Wash well in several changes of distilled water for 2 minutes.
4 Differentiate in the appropriate hydrochloric acid solution (see above) for 3 minutes.
5 Treat with potassium permaganate solution for 1 minute.
6 Wash in several changes of distilled water for 2 minutes.
7 Dehydrate, clear and mount in DPX (for tubercle bacilli) *or* blot dry, clear in xylene and mount in DPX (for leprosy bacilli).
8 Examine by fluorescence microscopy (see note 1).

Results

Tubercle and leprosy bacilli	golden-yellow (see note below)
Background	dark green

Notes

1 The use of a K530 barrier filter is recommended for this method.
2 This method is highly recommended as a screening technique particularly when organisms are likely to be scanty.

CHROMOTROPE–ANILINE BLUE (for collagen and Mallory bodies (alcoholic hyalin))

Reference: Churg J., Prado A. (1956) *Archives of Pathology* **62**, 505

Solutions

Celestine blue solution (see page 118)
Mayer's haematoxylin (see page 121)
1 per cent aqueous phosphomolybdic acid

Chromotrope–aniline blue solution
Dissolve 1.5 g aniline blue in 200 ml distilled water and 2.5 ml concentrated hydrochloric acid using gentle heat (50°C). Then add 6 g chromotrope 2R. The pH of this solution is approximately 1.0.

Technique

1   Take control section and test section to distilled water.
2   Stain in celestine blue solution for 5 minutes.
3   Rinse briefly in distilled water for 30 seconds.
4   Stain in Mayer's haematoxylin for 5 minutes.
5   Wash in distilled water for 1–2 minutes.
6   Treat with 1 per cent phosphomolybdic acid for 1–3 minutes.
7   Rinse in distilled water for 30 seconds.
8   Stain in chromotrope–aniline blue solution for 8 minutes.
9   Rinse in distilled water for 30 seconds.
10 Blot.
11 Dehydrate rapidly, clear and mount.

Results

Collagen   blue
Mallory bodies   greyish blue, sometimes red
Giant mitochondria   red
Nuclei   blue-black

Notes

1 The use of an iron haematoxylin sequence is necessary because of the acidity of the chromotrope–aniline blue solution.
2 Weigert's haematoxylin can be used as an alternative nuclear stain.
3 Some batches of celestine blue may prove to be unsuitable.

GORDON AND SWEETS' RETICULIN TECHNIQUE

Reference: Gordon H., Sweets H.H. (1936) *American Journal of Pathology* **12**, 545

Solutions

5 per cent aqueous oxalic acid
2 per cent aqueous ferric ammonium sulphate (iron alum)

Acidified potassium permanganate
0.25 per cent aqueous potassium permanganate	47.5 ml
3 per cent aqueous sulphuric acid	2.5 ml

(Best prepared fresh before use.)

Ammoniacal silver solution (see page 114)

0.1 per cent aqueous yellow gold chloride
10 per cent formalin in tap water
5 per cent aqueous sodium thiosulphate ('hypo')

Technique

1 Section to distilled water.
2 Treat section with acidified potassium permanganate solution for 5 minutes.
3 Wash briefly in distilled water for 10 seconds.
4 Bleach with oxalic acid for 1–2 minutes.
5 Wash well in running tap water for 2 minutes.
6 Wash in several changes of distilled water for 30 seconds.
7 Treat section with iron alum solution for 5 minutes.
8 Wash in several changes of distilled water for 1 minute.
9 Treat with ammoniacal silver solution for 20 seconds (see notes below).
10 Wash in distilled water for 10 seconds.

11	Treat with 10 per cent formalin for 1 minute to reduce silver salts.
12	Wash well in running tap water for 2 minutes.
13	Tone in gold chloride solution for 2 minutes. *This step is optional.*
14	Wash in several changes of distilled water for 2 minutes.
15	Treat with 'hypo' solution for 3 minutes.
16	Wash well in running tap water for 2 minutes.
17	Dehydrate, clear and mount.

Results

Reticulin	black
Collagen	yellow brown in the untoned section, grey or black after toning
Background	clear

Notes

1 Store the ammoniacal silver solution at 4°C. This solution keeps for several weeks.
2 Agitation of the section when treating with the silver solution and the formalin solution improves the results.
3 The time required in the ammoniacal silver solution will vary depending on the ambient temperature, whether the specimen has been decalcified and the potency of the silver solution.
4 Counterstaining in 1 per cent aqueous neutral red, if desired, can be carried out *after* the treatment with 'hypo'.

GRIMELIUS SILVER METHOD FOR ARGYROPHIL CELLS

Reference:Grimelius L. (1968) *Acta Societa Medica Uppsala* 73, 243

Solutions

(a)   *Silver solution*

Acetate buffer (pH 5.6)	10 ml
Redistilled water	87 ml
1 per cent aqueous silver nitrate (fresh)	3 ml

(b)   *Reducing solution*

Hydroquinone	1 g
Sodium sulphite crystals	5 g
Distilled water	100 ml

(Freshly prepared)

Technique

1   Take test section and control section to distilled water.
2   Transfer sections to preheated silver solution in a water bath at 60°C for 3 hours.
3   Remove sections from the silver solution and drain thoroughly.
4   Place sections in the freshly prepared reducing solution in a water bath at 45°C for 1 minute.
5   Rinse sections in distilled water for 1 minute.
6   Examine the sections microscopically to check impregnation. If the sections are under-impregnated return to the silver bath for a further 5–10 minutes.
7   Drain the sections and repeat reduction.
8   Rinse in distilled water for 1 minute.
9   Wash well in running tap water for 5 minutes.
10   Dehydrate, clear and mount.

Results

Argyrophil cells	brown–black

Notes

1   This method gives very good results on freshly formalin-fixed A cells of the pancreatic islets. Carcinoid tumours will also give good results.
2   A light counterstain can be employed after completion of the reducing step. Light green (0.5 per cent aqueous) is recommended.

GROCOTT'S HEXAMINE-SILVER
(for fungi)

Reference: Grocott R.G. (1955). *American Journal of Clinical Pathology* 25,975

Solutions

5 per cent aqueous chromium trioxide (chromic acid)
1 per cent aqueous sodium metabisulphite
0.2 per cent aqueous gold chloride
5 per cent aqueous sodium thiosulphate ("hypo")
0.2 per cent light green in 1 per cent acetic acid

Stock hexamine-silver solution
To 100ml of 3 per cent aqueous hexamine add 5 ml of 5 per cent silver nitrate. The white precipitate which forms will dissolve on shaking. The solution will keep for at least 1-2 months at 4°C.

Working solution
Dilute 2ml of freshly prepared 5 per cent aqueous sodium tetraborate (borax) solution with 25ml of distilled water. Mix well and add 25ml of stock hexamine-silver solution. Mix well.

Technique

1   Take test section and control section to distilled water.
2   Treat sections with chromic acid solution for 1 hour at room temperature.
3   Wash well with distilled water for 2 minutes.
4   Bleach sections with the metabisulphite solution for 1 minute.
5   Wash well in running tap water for 5 minutes.
6   Wash well in several changes of distilled water for 2 minutes.
7   Place sections in pre-heated hexamine-silver solution in a Coplin jar at 56°C; this is best carried out in a water bath. Examine the sections after 10 minutes and then at 5 minute intervals until the fungi are blackened and the background is clear (see notes below).
8   Wash sections in several changes of distilled water for 2 minutes.

9 Treat sections with gold chloride solution for 2 minutes.
10 Wash in several changes of distilled water for 3 minutes.
11 Treat sections with "hypo" solution for 3 minutes.
12 Wash well in running tap water for 5 minutes.
13 Stain with light green solution for 30 seconds.
14 Wash in running tap water for 1 minute.
15 Dehydrate, clear and mount.

Results

Fungi, some mucins, glycogen	black
Background	green

Notes

1 This is the method of choice for demonstrating fungi.
2 *Pneumocystis carinii* is also well demonstrated by this method.
3 Although the method is time-consuming it very rarely fails to demonstrate fungi.
4 Impregnation of sections is critical. When the fungi appear dark brown the sections should be removed from the hexamine-silver solution.
5 Do not preheat the hexamine-silver solution for longer than 30 minutes as this will cause precipitation of silver on the sides of the Coplin jar.

HAEMATOXYLIN AND EOSIN
(for paraffin sections)

Solutions

Harris's haematoxylin (see page 120)
1 per cent aqueous eosin ws yellowish
2 per cent aqueous sodium bicarbonate
1 per cent hydrochloric acid in 70 per cent alcohol

Technique

1　Sections to water (see page 69).
2　Stain sections with Harris's haematoxylin for 10 minutes.
3　Wash well in running tap water for 3 minutes.
4　Differentiate the sections in acid alcohol for 10 seconds.
5　Wash sections in running tap water for 2 minutes.
6　'Blue' sections in 2 per cent sodium bicarbonate for 30 seconds.
7　Wash well in running tap water for 3 minutes.
8　Stain sections with 1 per cent eosin for 5 minutes.
9　Wash briefly in running tap water for 30 seconds.
10　Differentiate and dehydrate in graded alcohols (see notes on page 70).
11　Clear and mount.

Results

Nuclei   blue
Background   shades of pink to red

Notes

1　If other types of haematoxylin are used it may be necessary to stain the
　　sections for a longer time.
2　As a general rule, for every minute a section is in haematoxylin one second
　　is required in acid alcohol for differentiation.
3　It is advisable to add a crystal of phenol or thymol to the stock eosin
　　solution to prevent moulds from growing. Always filter the eosin prior to
　　use.

4   After the section has been 'blued' in sodium bicarbonate it is advisable to examine it microscopically to check nuclear staining before continuing with the rest of the technique.

HAEMATOXYLIN AND EOSIN (for fresh cryostat sections)

Solutions

As for paraffin sections.

Technique

1   Fix cryostat sections in 10 per cent aqueous formalin for 1–2 minutes.
2   Wash sections briefly in running tap water for 30 seconds.
3   Stain sections in Harris's haematoxylin for 1 minute.
4   Wash sections in running tap water for 30 seconds.
5   Differentiate sections in acid alcohol for 1–2 seconds.
6   Wash in running tap water and 'blue' in sodium bicarbonate for 10 seconds.
7   Wash well in running tap water for 30 seconds.
8   Stain with eosin for 20 seconds.
9   Wash briefly in running tap water for 10 seconds.
10   Dehydrate, clear and mount.

Results

Nuclei	blue
Background	shades of pink to red

Notes

1   Extra care must be taken when staining cryostat section as they have a tendency to lift off the slide.

JONES HEXAMINE-SILVER TECHNIQUE
(for glomerular basement membrane)

Reference: Jones D.B. (1957) *American Journal of Pathology* 33,313

Solutions

1 per cent aqueous periodic acid

Stock hexamine-silver solution
See Grocott's hexamine-silver solution (page 82)

Working hexamine-silver solution
See Grocott's hexamine-silver solution (page 82)

0.1 per cent aqueous gold chloride
5 per cent aqueous sodium thiosulphate ("hypo")
0.2 per cent light green in 1 per cent acetic acid

Technique

1　Take section to distilled water.
2　Treat with periodic acid solution for 10 minutes.
3　Wash well in several changes of distilled water for 2 minutes.
4　Place sections in preheated hexamine-silver solution in a Coplin jar at 56°C. This is best carried out in a water bath. Examine the sections after 15 minutes and then at 5 minute intervals until the basement membranes are blackened; this will take from 25-40 minutes.
5　Wash section in several changes of distilled water for 2 minutes.
6　Treat section with gold chloride solution for 2 minutes.
7　Wash well in distilled water for 1 minute.
8　Treat sections with "hypo" for 3 minutes.
9　Wash well in running tap water for 2 minutes.
10　Stain in light green solution for 30 seconds.
11　Wash briefly in running tap water for 30 seconds.
12　Dehydrate, clear and mount.

Results

Basement membranes (basal lamina) black
Background   green

Notes

1 This method is a modification of Grocott's method (page 82).
2 Best results are seen with sections which have been cut at 2μm.
3 Do not preheat the hexamine-silver solution for longer than 30 minutes as this will cause precipitation of silver onto the sides of the Coplin jar.
4 The haematoxylin and eosin stain can be used in place of the light green.
5 This method may require modification when used on resin sections.

LINDER'S TECHNIQUE FOR PERIPHERAL NERVE IN PARAFFIN SECTIONS

Reference: Linder J.E. (1978) *Journal of Anatomy* **127**, 543

Solutions

(a) *Buffer stock solution*
Collidine	6.6 ml
Distilled water	450 ml

Adjust to PH 7.2–7.4 with 10 per cent nitric acid and make up to a total volume of 500 ml with distilled water

(b) *Buffer working solution*
Stock solution	8 ml
Distilled water	92 ml

(c) *Impregnating solution*
Distilled water (heated to 60°C)	84 ml
1 per cent aqueous silver nitrate	4 ml
0.38 per cent aqueous sodium cyanate	4 ml
Buffer stock solution	8 ml

Add the ingredients in the order listed, mixing well with each addition.

(d) *Physical developer stock solution*
Sodium sulphite ($Na_2 SO_3.7H_2O$)	20 g
Sodium tetraborate	4.75 g
Distilled water	450 ml

Heat the solution to 50°C and add 10 g leaf gelatin.

(e) *Physical developer working solution*
Stock solution	95 ml
2 per cent aqueous hydroquinone	5 ml
1 per cent aqueous silver nitrate	2 ml

Technique

1 Take sections to absolute alcohol.
2 Celloidinise sections (see page 71).
3 Wash in distilled water for 2 minutes.
4 Place sections in diluted buffer solution (b). Soft tissues 10–20 minutes at 60°C; decalcified tissues overnight at 45°C.
5 Drain and transfer sections to the silver impregnating solution (c); soft tissue 10–30 minutes at 60°C; decalcified tissue 90 minutes at 45°C.
6 Wash well in several changes of distilled water for 3 minutes.
7 Place sections into the physical developer working solution (e) at approximately 25°C. This stage must be controlled microscopically. Optimum results are usually seen after 5 minutes.
8 Wash well in distilled water.
9 Dehydrate, clear and mount.

Results

Nerve fibres and neurendocrine granules   black

Notes

1 This method is highly recommended for nerve fibres of the peripheral nervous sytem.
2 It is very important to stir the physical developer solution constantly during preparation, as a white precipitate will otherwise form.

MALLORY'S PHOSPHOTUNGSTIC ACID HAEMATOXYLIN (PTAH)

Reference: Mallory F.B. (1900) *Journal of Experimental Medicine* **5**, 15
Shum M.W.K., Hon J.K.Y. (1969) *Journal of Medical Laboratory Technology* **26**, 38

Solutions

0.25 per cent aqueous potassium permanganate
5 per cent aqueous oxalic acid
Phosphotungstic acid haematoxylin solution (see page 123)

Technique

1 Section to distilled water.
2 Treat with potassium permanganate solution for 5 minutes.
3 Wash in distilled water for 20 seconds.
4 Bleach with oxalic acid solution for 1 minute.
5 Wash well in running tap water for 2 minutes.
6 Wash in distilled water for 20 seconds.
7 Stain with PTAH solution (in a Coplin jar) for 12–14 hours at room temperature.
8 Wash in distilled water for 20 seconds.
9 Dehydrate, clear and mount.

Results

Muscle, keratin, erythrocytes, cilia, myelin, nuclei, Paneth cell granules, oncocytes	blue
Collagen and reticulin	brick red

Notes

1 The Shum and Hon modification of Mallory's original technique is highly recommended because it gives a more reproducible result.

2 More precise results are seen by staining at room temperature than by staining at 56°C for 4 hours.

3 The haematoxylin solution can be used repeatedly until staining deterioration is observed. The stain should be filtered before use.

MASSON–FONTANA TECHNIQUE FOR MELANIN

Reference: Fontana A. (1912) *Dermatologische Wochenschrift* **55**, 1003
Masson P. (1914) *Comptes Rendus Hebdomadaires des Seances de l'Academie des Sciences* **158**, 59

Solutions

Fontana's silver solution (see page 119)
0.5 per cent aqueous sodium thiosulphate ('hypo')
1 per cent aqueous neutral red

Technique

1   Take the test section and the control section to distilled water.
2   Filter the Fontana's silver solution into a thoroughly cleaned Coplin jar and place the sections in it. Cover the jar with aluminium foil to make it light proof.
3   Either place the Coplin jar in the 56°C oven for 20–40 minutes or leave overnight at room temperature.
4   Wash the sections in several changes of distilled water for 1 minute.
5   Check the control section microscopically to see if the melanin is positive
6   Treat sections with 0.5 per cent 'hypo' for not longer than 2 minutes.
7   Wash in running tap water for 2 minutes.
8   Counterstain in the neutral red solution for 5 minutes.
9   Wash in tap water for 1 minute.
10   Dehydrate, clear and mount.

Results

Melanin   black
Nuclei   red

Notes

1 It is important to note that other pigments will also reduce the silver solution but melanin invariably gives a positive reaction in a shorter time. Enterochromaffin and some lipofuscins will reduce the silver solution but this usually takes longer than 24 hours at room temperature.

2 A weak solution of 'hypo' is used in this technique as stronger solutions tend to bleach the reduced silver.

MILLER'S STAIN FOR ELASTIC FIBRES

Reference: Miller P.J. (1971) *Medical Laboratory Technology* 28, 148

Solutions

0.5 per cent aqueous potassium permanganate
1 per cent aqueous oxalic acid
Miller's elastic stain (see page 122)
van Gieson's stain (see page 125)

Technique

1   Sections to water.
2   Treat with potassium permanganate for 5 minutes.
3   Wash in water.
4   Bleach sections with oxalic acid for 2 minutes.
5   Wash well in running tap water.
6   Wash in several changes of 95 per cent alcohol.
7   Place the section in a Coplin jar containing either (a) undiluted stain for 1–3 hours or (b) stain diluted with equal parts of 95 per cent alcohol for 12–18 hours.
8   Wash in 95 per cent alcohol to remove excess stain.
9   Wash well in running tap water for 2 minutes.
10 Counterstain in van Gieson's stain for 2 minutes.
11 Dehydrate, clear and mount.

Results

Elastic fibres	black
Muscle	yellow
Collagen	red

Notes

1 The overnight staining method gives crisper results.
2 If preferred the haematoxylin and eosin stain can be used in place of the van Gieson stain.

OIL RED O TECHNIQUE FOR LIPIDS

Reference: Lillie R.D., Ashburn L.L. (1943) *Archives of Pathology* **36**, 432

Solutions

Oil Red O Stock solution
Dissolve 0.5 g oil red O in 200 ml isopropyl alcohol in a large flask, in a 56°C water bath, for 1 hour.

Oil Red O working solution
Make this solution before use by adding 4 parts of distilled water to 6 parts of stock solution. Mix well and allow to stand for 10 minutes. Filter using a fine filter paper (Whatman No 42).

Mayer's haematoxylin (see page 121)
60 per cent isopropyl alcohol

Technique

1   Rinse frozen sections in distilled water.
2   Rinse in 60 per cent isopropyl alcohol.
3   Stain the sections in the oil red O working solution for 10 minutes.
4   Wash sections briefly in 60 per cent isopropyl alcohol until excess dye is removed.
5   Wash well in distilled water for 2 minutes.
6   Stain nuclei in Mayer's haematoxylin for 1 minute.
7   Wash in distilled water for 1 minute.
8   'Blue' in 2 per cent sodium bicarbonate for 30 seconds.
9   Wash in tap water for 2 minutes.
10 Mount in an aqueous mountant.

Results

Lipids   red
Nuclei   blue

Notes

The handling of loose frozen sections is quite difficult for inexperienced workers. Cryostat sections tend to be more easily handled. The use of slides coated with gelatin will help to keep the sections on the slide.

The loose frozen sections can be picked up on to gelatinised slides either prior to or after completion of staining.

Do not mount sections in a xylene based mountant as this will dissolve the stained lipid.

MODIFIED ORCEIN TECHNIQUE FOR HEPATITIS B SURFACE ANTIGEN

Reference: Shikata T, Uzawa T, Yoshiwara N, Akatsuka T, Yamazaki S (1974) *Japanese Journal of Experimental Medicine* **44**, 25

Solutions

(a) *Acidified potassium permanganate*
0.25 per cent aqueous potassium permanganate   95 ml
3 per cent aqueous sulphuric acid   5 ml
   Mix well. Store at room temperature.
(b) *1 per cent aqueous oxalic acid*
(c) *Orcein solution*
Orcein (synthetic)   1 g
70 per cent alcohol   100 ml
Hydrochloric acid 'analytical grade'
(concentrated)   2 ml
(d) 1 per cent hydrochloric acid in 70 per cent alcohol

Technique

1   Take the test section and control section to distilled water.
2   Treat sections with acidified potassium permanganate for 15 minutes.
3   Bleach sections with 1 per cent oxalic acid for 3 minutes.
4   Wash in several changes of distilled water for 2 minutes.
5   Stain sections in a Coplin jar containing the orcein solution for 2–4 hours at room temperature.
6   Rinse in distilled water for 30 seconds.
7   Differentiate in acid alcohol, checking the control section microscopically for correct staining.
8   Dehydrate, clear and mount.

Results

HBs antigen, elastic fibres and copper associated protein	dark brown
Background	clear to light brown

Notes

1. Certain batches of synthetic orcein may give poor staining.
2. Shorter staining times in orcein can be employed by raising the temperature of the stain to 37°C or 56°C. The best results are seen by staining for a longer period at room temperature.
3. The acidified potassium permanganate solution can have a short shelf life. It may be necessary to make this solution fresh each time before use.

PERIODIC ACID–SCHIFF TECHNIQUE (PAS)

References: Schiff U. (1866) *Justus Liebig's Annalen der Chemie* **140**, 92
McManus J.F.A. (1946) *Nature* **158**, 202

Solutions

1 per cent aqueous periodic acid
Schiff's reagent (see page 124)
Carazzi's haematoxylin (see page 116)
2 per cent aqueous sodium bicarbonate
1 per cent hydrochloric acid in 70 per cent alcohol

Technique

1   Take the test section and control section to distilled water.
2   Treat with periodic acid solution for 10 minutes.
3   Wash in distilled water for 30 seconds.
4   Treat with Schiff's reagent for 20 minutes.
5   Wash well in running tap water for 10 minutes (this will intensify the colour reaction).
6   Stain the nuclei with Carazzi's haematoxylin for 2 minutes.
7   Wash in running tap water for 2 minutes.
8   Differentiate, if necessary, in acid alcohol.
9   Wash in running tap water for 2 minutes.
10 'Blue', if necessary, in sodium bicarbonate solution for 1 minute.
11 Wash briefly in running tap water for 30 seconds.
12 Dehydrate, clear and mount.

Results

PAS positive material	magenta
Nuclei	blue

Notes

1   Although this method is easy and simple to perform, a poor batch of Schiff's reagent (see page 124) often leads to poor results

2 This technique will positively demonstrate many substances in tissue sections and it is advisable to set up the correct control section (e.g. for mucin, use a control section of jejunum).

3 The demonstration of glycogen can be made highly selective if amylase (diastase) digestion is used on a duplicate section (see below).

AMYLASE (DIASTASE)–PAS

Solutions

1 per cent aqueous malt diastase
Other solutions are under PAS technique (see page 100)

Technique

1 Take two test sections and two control sections to distilled water.

2 Treat one test section and one control section with 1 per cent aqueous malt diastase in a Coplin jar for 1 hour at 37°C.

3 Wash well in running tap water for 10 minutes.

4 Rinse in distilled water for 1 minute.

5 Treat all sections with periodic acid, Schiff's reagent and haematoxylin in the usual way (see page 100).

6 Dehydrate, clear and mount.

Results

Glycogen   magenta red in the non-diastase section only
Nuclei   blue

Notes

1 The diastase digestion will make this technique highly selective for glycogen.

2 The control section of choice is rabbit liver which has been fixed in alcoholic picric acid.

3 It is advisable to test each new batch of amylase (diastase) before use in order to work out the correct digestion time.

PERLS' PRUSSIAN BLUE REACTION
(for haemosiderin and ferric iron salts)

Reference: Perls M.(1867) *Virchows Archiv für pathologische Anatomie und Physiologie und für klinische Medizin* **39, 42**

Solutions

2 per cent aqueous hydrochloric acid
2 per cent aqueous potassium ferrocyanide
1 per cent aqueous neutral red

Technique

1 Take the test section and control section to water.
2 Mix equal parts 2 per cent hydrochloric acid and 2 per cent potassium ferrocyanide, then filter the mixture on to the sections. Leave for 15 minutes.
3 Wash sections in several changes of distilled water for 1 minute.
4 Stain sections with 1 per cent neutral red for 5 minutes.
5 Wash sections in running tap water for 30 seconds.
6 Dehydrate and differentiate in alcohol, clear and mount.

Results

Haemosiderin (ferric iron salts)   blue
Nuclei   red
Background   pale red

Notes

1 If possible analytical grade chemicals should be used.
2 The technique is best carried out at room temperature as raised temperatures (56°C) can give rise to false positive results.
3 Thorough washing of the sections with distilled water after treatment with the acid–ferrocyanide solution is necessary, as a heavy precipitate can form on the sections after staining with neutral red. This is due to a reaction between any excess acid–ferrocyanide still present in the section and the neutral red.
4 It is advisable to change the stock solution of potassium ferrocyanide every 8 weeks as it slowly deteriorates and will give rise to artefactual blue granules.

MODIFIED RHODANINE TECHNIQUE FOR COPPER

Reference: Lindquist R.R. (1969) *Archives of Pathology* **87, 370**

Solutions

(a)   *Rhodanine stock solution*

5-para-dimethylaminobenzylidene rhodanine	0.2 g
Absolute alcohol	100 ml

(b)   *Rhodanine working solution*

Stock rhodanine solution	3.0 ml
Distilled water	7.0 ml

(Shake the stock rhodanine solution *well* before use.)

(c)   Carazzi's haematoxylin (see page 116)

(d)   *Borax solution*

Disodium tetraborate	0.5 g
Distilled water	100 ml

Technique

1   Take test solution and control solution to distilled water.
2   Stain in the rhodanine working solution for 3 hours at 56°C.
3   Wash in several changes of distilled water for 3 minutes.
4   Stain with Carazzi's haematoxylin for 3 minutes.
5   Wash in distilled water for 30 seconds.
6   Treat with borax solution for 10 seconds.
7   Wash well in several changes of distilled water for 3 minutes.
8   Dehydrate, clear and mount.

Results

Copper	red
Nuclei	light blue
Bile, if present in section	green

Notes

1. Control material is best obtained from livers of patients suffering from Wilson's disease, primary biliary cirrhosis or other forms of chronic cholestasis.
2. Certain synthetic mountants will cause fading of the stained copper. The most acceptable mountant is DPX.

THIOFLAVINE T TECHNIQUE FOR AMYLOID

Reference: Vassar P.S., Culling F.A. (1959) *Archives of Pathology* **68**, 487

Solutions

1 per cent aqueous thioflavine T (freshly prepared)
Mayer's or Carazzi's haematoxylin (see pages 121 and 116)
1 per cent aqueous acetic acid

Technique

1 Take test section and control section to water.
2 Stain the sections with either Mayer's or Carazzi's haematoxylin for 2 minutes (this masks the nuclear fluorescence).
3 Wash well in running tap water.
4 Stain the sections with thioflavine T for 5 minutes.
5 Differentiate the excess thioflavine T in 1 per cent acetic acid for 10–15 minutes.
6 Wash well in running tap water for 2 minutes.
7 Blot dry.
8 Dehydrate and clear in fresh alcohol and xylene.
9 Mount in DPX mountant.
10 Examine by fluorescence microscopy.

Results

Depending on the types of filter used in the fluorescence microscope, amyloid can be seen stained either silver-white or yellow.

Notes

1. It is advisable to prepare the thioflavine T solution shortly before use.
2. Certain mountants will exhibit autofluorescence, e.g. Canada balsam.
3. The use of pots of dehydrating and clearing agents previously used for other staining techniques should be avoided. The reason is that dyes such as eosin may contaminate the section and will impart non-specific fluorescence to the section.

MODIFIED VON KOSSA TECHNIQUE FOR OSTEOID SEAMS

Reference: Tripp E.J., MacKay E.H. (1972) *Stain Technology* **47**, 129

Solutions

2 per cent aqueous silver nitrate

Reducing solution

Sodium hypophosphite	5 g
0.1 M sodium hydroxide	0.2 ml
Distilled water	100 ml

5 per cent aqueous sodium thiosulphate ('hypo')
10 per cent aqueous formic acid
Haematoxylin and eosin (see page 84) or van Gieson's stain (see page 125)

Technique

1 Take thin blocks (2 mm) of bone fixed in 90 per cent alcohol or 10 per cent neutral buffered formalin for 2 days.
2 If formalin fixed wash well in several changes of large volumes of distilled water (see notes below) for 2 hours.
3 Place the tissue block in 2 per cent aqueous silver nitrate for 2–4 days at room temperature in a light proof container (see notes below).
4 Wash well in several changes of distilled water for 1 hour (see notes below).
5 Wash in running tap water for 1 hour.
6 Treat with the reducing solution for 2 days at room temperature.
7 Wash in running tap water for 1 hour.
8 Treat with 5 per cent 'hypo' for 24 hours.
9 Wash in running tap water for 1 hour.
10 Decalcify in 10 per cent formic acid.

11 Check decalcification daily using the chemical test (see page 125).
12 Paraffin process the decalcified tissue.
13 Cut (5–8 μm) sections and mount on slides using a plasma adhesive.
14 Dry sections at 56°C for 1 hour.
15 Take sections to distilled water.
16 Stain sections with either the haematoxylin and eosin technique (see page 84) or van Gieson's method (see page 125).
17 Dehydrate, clear and mount.

Results

Mineralised bone	black
Osteoid seams	pink (with H & E)
	red (with van Gieson)
Bone marrow	yellow (with van Gieson)
	pinks (with H & E)

Notes

1 Alcohol fixation is recommended for this technique.
2 The washing of the tissue blocks in large volumes of distilled water is best carried out using an automatic tissue processor (with agitation).
3 The impregnation of the tissue blocks can be carried out in a suitably cleaned glass container completely covered with aluminium foil. The volume of silver nitrate used should be at least 20 times that of the tissue block.
4 By using a slight modification of this technique the time in silver nitrate solution can be shortened to 24 hours. This modification (Phillpotts C.J. 1980, personal communication) utilises 3 per cent silver nitrate in 80 per cent alcohol at 37°C for 24 hours. The reducing solution is also used at 37°C but only for 24 hours.

MODIFIED ZIEHL–NEELSEN FOR LEPROSY BACILLI

References: Faraco J. (1938) *Revista Braziliera de Leprologia* **6,** 77
Fite G.L., Cambre P.J., Turner M.H. (1947) *Archives of Pathology* **43,** 624

Solutions

As for the standard Ziehl–Neelson method (see page 112)

Technique

1 Warm the test section and the control section and deparaffinise in a mixture of two parts xylene to one part vegetable oil preheated to 56°C. Leave for 10 minutes.
2 Blot sections dry and wash in running tap water. Repeat this step if any xylene–oil mixture is left on the section.
3 Filter the carbol fuchsin on to the slides and leave for 30 minutes. **Do not heat.**
4 Wash in running tap water for 5 minutes.
5 Differentiate in 1 per cent acid alcohol for 2 minutes.
6 Wash in running tap water for 5 minutes.
7 Counterstain with Harris's haematoxylin or 0.1 per aqueous methylene blue for 30 seconds.
8 Wash well in tap water.
9 Blot sections dry and clear in xylene. This step may have to be repeated until the sections are completely clear.
10 Mount.

Results

Leprosy bacilli	red
Nuclei	blue

Notes

1 When blotting the sections use the best quality blotting paper, which should be smooth and fluff-free.
2 Avoid over exposure with the acid alcohol as leprosy bacilli are less acid and alcohol-fast than tubercle bacilli.
3 Do not overstain with either haematoxylin or methylene blue solutions.
4 After differentiation with acid alcohol it is advisable to check the control section microscopically to see if the leprosy bacilli are easily visible.

ZIEHL–NEELSEN TECHNIQUE FOR TUBERCLE BACILLI

References: Ziehl F. (1882) *Deutsche medizinische Wochenschrift* 8, 451
Neelsen F. (1883) *Zentralblatt für die medizinischen Wissenschaften* 21, 497

Solutions

Carbol fuchsin solution (see page 117)
1 per cent hydrochloric acid in 70 per cent alcohol
Harris's haematoxylin (see page 120)

Technique

1 Take the test section and the control section to water.
2 Filter the carbol fuchsin solution on to the sections and gently heat until steam rises from the solution. The solution is left on the section for 10 minutes with occasional heating.
3 Wash the sections in running tap water for 5 minutes.
4 Differentiate in 1 per cent acid alcohol for approximately 10 minutes. Check the control section microscopically to see if differentiation is correct.
5 Wash well in running tap water for 5 minutes.
6 Counterstain with Harris's haematoxylin for 1 minute.
7 Wash well in running tap water for 5 minutes.
8 Dehydrate, clear and mount.

Results

Tubercle bacilli   red
Nuclei   blue

Notes

1 The counterstain should be light as the haematoxylin can mask the tubercle bacilli.
2 Carbol fuchsin solutions deteriorate with age.
3 The staining of tubercle bacilli can be carried out using the carbol fuchsin solution in a Coplin jar at 56°C for 30 minutes.
4 0.1 per cent aqueous methylene blue can be used as an alternative counterstain.

SOLUTIONS

AMMONIACAL SILVER SOLUTION FOR GORDON AND SWEETS' TECHNIQUE

Reference: Gordon H., Sweets, H.H. (1936) *American Journal of Pathology* **12**, 545

Reagents

10 per cent aqueous silver nitrate	5 ml
3.1 per cent aqueous sodium hydroxide	5 ml
Concentrated ammonia	

Place 5 ml of 10 per cent aqueous silver nitrate in a thoroughly cleaned 100 ml flask. Add concentrated ammonia drop by drop until the precipitate formed just redissolves (see notes below). Add 5 ml of 3.1 per cent aqueous sodium hydroxide and mix well. The precipitate which forms will gradually dissolve upon further addition of ammonia as before. The titration should be complete when only a few precipitate granules remain in the solution. Make up to a final volume of 5 ml with distilled water. Store the solution in a dark bottle at 4°C. Filter before use.

Notes

1   The secret of a good ammoniacal silver solution is in the titration with ammonia. When adding ammonia drop by drop make sure that the drops used are small. The addition of excess ammonia at either stage of titration will give rise to poorly sensitive silver solution.
2   Ammoniacal silver solutions can be explosive if kept in direct sunlight.

AURAMINE–RHODAMINE SOLUTION

Reference: Silver A., Sonnenwirth A.C., Alex N. (1966) *Journal of Clinical Pathology* **19**, 583

Reagents

Auramine O	1.5 g
Rhodamine B	0.75 g
Distilled water	50 ml
Glycerol	75 ml
Liquefied phenol (melted at 56°C)	10 ml

Add 1.5 g auramine O and 0.75 g rhodamine B to 50 ml distilled water and 75 ml glycerol. Mix well, and add 10 ml liquefied phenol. Heat the mixture in a 56°C oven or water bath to help dissolve the dyes. This solution will keep for about 2–3 months.

Notes

1 Care must be taken when handling the two dyes and the phenol because of their toxicity.

CARAZZI'S HAEMATOXYLIN

Reference: Carazzi D. (1911) *Zeitschrift für wissenschaftliche Mikroskopie und für mikroskopische Technik* **28**, 275

Reagents

Haematoxylin	1 g
Glycerol	200 ml
Potassium or ammonium alum	50 g
Distilled water	800 ml
Potassium iodate	0.2 g

Dissolve the haematoxylin in the glycerol. Dissolve the alum in about 700 ml of the distilled water at room temperature. This will take at least 24 hours before all the alum goes into solution.

Mix the haematoxylin and the alum solutions gradually in small amounts, shaking the mixture well. Dissolve the potassium iodate in the remaining volume of distilled water and then add to the haematoxylin–alum solution. Mix the solution thoroughly, then filter. This solution is ready for immediate use and keeps well.

CARBOL FUCHSIN SOLUTION FOR ZIEHL–NEELSEN METHOD

Reference: Ziehl F. (1882) *Deutsche medizinische Wochenschrift* 8, 451
Neelsen F. (1883) *Zentralblatt für die medizinischen Wissenschaften* 21, 497

Reagents

Basic fuchsin (coarsely granular)	1 g
Ethyl alcohol	10 ml
Phenol	5 g
Distilled water	100 ml

Dissolve 1 g basic fuchsin (see notes below) in 10 ml ethyl alcohol. Dissolve 5 g phenol in 100 ml distilled water. Mix the two solutions together. Filter and store.

Notes

1 The coarsely granular form of basic fuchsin gives better results than the more purified form as used in Schiff's reagent.
2 Care must be taken when handling phenol as this can cause skin burning.

CELESTINE BLUE SOLUTION

Reference: Gray P., Pickle F.M., Muser M.D., Hayweiser J. (1956) *Stain Technology* **31**, 141

Reagents

Celestine blue B or R	1 g
Sulphuric acid (concentrated)	0.5 ml
2.5 per cent aqueous ferric ammonium sulphate (iron alum) solution	86 ml
Glycerol	1.4 ml

Grind the celestine blue to a paste with the sulphuric acid and then gradually add the iron alum solution with constant mixing. Add the glycerol, mix and place in a 56°C oven to dissolve. Cool and filter. It is advisable to filter again prior to use.

FONTANA'S AMMONIACAL SILVER SOLUTION

Reference: Fontana A. (1912) *Dermatologische Wochenschrift* **55**, 1003
Masson P. (1914) *Comptes Rendus Hebdomadaires des Seances de l'Academie des Sciences* **158**, 59

Reagents

10 per cent aqueous silver nitrate	20 ml
Distilled water	20 ml
Concentrated ammonia	

In a thoroughly clean 100 ml flask place 20 ml 10 per cent aqueous silver nitrate. Add concentrated ammonia drop by drop until the formed precipitate almost dissolves leaving a faint opalescence. If too much ammonia is added then a few drops of silver nitrate solution will restore the faint opalescence to the solution. Add 20 ml distilled water, mix and filter. Store in a dark container at 4°C.

Notes

1   As with all ammoniacal silver solutions the titration with ammonia is critical. Small drops of ammonia should be used and the solution should be thoroughly shaken and mixed between each drop.
2   The ammoniacal silver solution has potential explosive properties if kept in direct sunlight.

HARRIS'S HAEMATOXYLIN

Reference: Harris H.F. (1900) *Journal of Applied Microscopic Laboratory Methods* **3**, 777

Reagents

Haematoxylin	5 g
Ethyl alcohol	50 ml
Potassium or ammonium alum	100 g
Distilled water	950 g
Mercuric oxide	2.5 g
Glacial acetic acid	40 ml

Dissolve the haematoxylin in the alcohol in the 56°C oven or water bath. Dissolve the alum in the distilled water using gentle heat over a Bunsen burner. Stir the alum solution frequently until completely dissolved. Add the alcoholic haematoxylin solution to the hot alum solution. Bring the mixture to the boil stirring frequently. Remove the haematoxylin–alum mixture from the Bunsen burner and add the mercuric oxide carefully and slowly (see notes below). Cool the solution quickly in a container of cold water; when cool add the acetic acid and filter. The solution is ready for immediate use but refiltering may be necessary.

Technique

1   Care must be taken when handling mercuric oxide because of its toxicity. If mercuric oxide is added to boiling haematoxylin–alum the solution will effervesce and spill. To prevent this choose a suitable large flask for the preparation of this solution. After boiling the solution of haematoxylin–alum, allow to cool slightly, then add the mercuric oxide carefully and slowly.

2   Mercuric oxide is also corrosive. This may cause corrosion of certain parts of staining machines etc.

MAYER'S HAEMATOXYLIN

Reference: Mayer P. (1903) *Zeitschrift für wissenschaftliche Mikroskopie und für mikroskopische Technik* **20**, 409

Reagents

Haematoxylin	1 g
Distilled water	1000 ml
Potasium or ammonium alum	50 g
Sodium iodate	0.2 g
Citric acid	1 g
Chloral hydrate	50 g

Dissolve the haematoxylin, alum and sodium iodate in the distilled water by leaving for 24 hours at room temperature. Add the chloral hydrate and citric acid, shake well and boil for 5 minutes. Cool and filter. Best results are seen if the solution is left to ripen for one week.

MILLER'S ELASTIC STAIN

Reference: Miller P.J. (1971) *Medical Laboratory Technology* 28, 148

Reagents

Victoria blue 4R	1 g
New fuchsin	1 g
Crystal violet	1 g
Distilled water	200 ml
Resorcinol	4 g
Dextrin	1 g
30 per cent aqueous ferric chloride (freshly prepared)	50 ml
95 per cent alcohol	200 ml
Hydrochloric acid (concentrated)	2ml

Heat 200 ml distilled water to about 60°C, then add the Victoria blue, new fuchsin and crystal violet. Shake well to dissolve. Then add resorcinol and shake well to dissolve, followed by the dextrin and the freshly prepared ferric chloride solution. Bring the mixture to the boil and filter whilst hot. Transfer the precipitate and the filter paper to the original container and redissolve the precipitate in 200 ml of 95 per cent alcohol. Boil for 15 minutes, cool and filter and make up volume with 95 per cent alcohol. Add 2 ml concentrated hydrochloric acid and store at room temperature. This stain can be used either in its concentrated form or diluted with equal parts 95 per cent alcohol.

Notes

1 Always use freshly prepared ferric chloride solution.
2 Extreme care must be taken when boiling the alcoholic solution.

PHOSPHOTUNGSTIC ACID HAEMATOXYLIN SOLUTION (MODIFIED)

Reference: Shum M.W.K, Hon J.K.Y. (1969) *Journal of Medical Laboratory Technology* **26**, 38

Reagents

Haematein	0.08 g
Phosphotungstic acid	0.9 g
Distilled water	100 ml

Grind 0.08 g haematein with 1 ml of distilled water in a pestle and mortar until a fine chocolate brown paste is produced (see notes below). Dissolve 0.9 g phosphotungstic acid in the remaining distilled water and mix with the ground haematein paste. Bring the solution to the boil, cool and filter.

Notes

1 Batches of haematein which are light brown or straw colour will prove unsatisfactory.
2 The proportion of haematein and phosphotungstic acid is important for good results.

SCHIFF'S REAGENT

References: Schiff U. (1866) *Justus Liebig's Annalen der Chemie* **140**, 92
de Thomasi J.A. (1936) *Stain Technology* **11**, 137

Reagents

Basic fuchsin (pararosanilene)	1 g
Distilled water	200 ml
Potassium or sodium metabisulphite	2 g
Hydrochloric acid 'analytical grade'	2 ml
Activated charcoal	2 g

Bring the distilled water to the boil, remove from heat, carefully and slowly add the basic fuchsin. Cool the mixture to 50°C, then add the metabisulphite. Mix well and cool the mixture to room temperature. Add the hydrochloric acid and the activated charcoal. Mix thoroughly and store in the dark at 4°C for 24 hours. Filter the solution and store in a dark container at 4°C. The filtered solution should be a pale straw colour. Storage of the solution for a prolonged period of time will cause it to turn pink. This is due to the loss of sulphur dioxide which results in the restoration of the basic fuchsin colour. If this happens the solution should be discarded.

Notes

1   Not all batches of basic fuchsin are suitable for making Schiff's reagent. Best results are usually obtained by using pararosanilene hydrochloride.
2   Experience has shown that an analytical grade of hydrochloric acid gives better results in the manufacture of Schiff's reagent.

VAN GIESON'S STAIN

References: van Gieson (1889) *New York Medical Journal* 50:57
Curtis F. (1905) *Archives de Médicine expérimentale et d'Anatomie Pathologique* 17:603

Reagents

Saturated aqueous picric acid	100 ml
1 per cent aqueous acid fuchsin	10 ml

Mix the two solutions together. Boil for 3 minutes, cool and filter.

Notes

1 Brighter staining which shows less fading can be obtained using the modification of Curtis (1905) which uses 10 ml of 1 per cent aqueous Ponceau S, 1 ml glacial acetic acid and 90 ml saturated aqueous picric acid.

Chemical test for end point decalcification

This is a simple method to detect the presence of calcium in decalcifying fluid. It is used when X-ray facilities are not available, or in some cases, unsuitable e.g. after fixation with mercury containing solutions, or after impregnation with silver salts as in the Tripp and Mackay method. Take 5 ml of decalcifying fluid and neutralize with strong ammonia, drop by drop, using pH paper. Add 5 ml aqueous saturated ammonium oxalate and mix well. Any turbidity present in the solution indicates the presence of calcium and the specimen should then be placed in fresh decalcifying solution. Decalcification is complete when after the addition of ammonia and ammonium oxalate the solution remains clear after 30 minutes.

Further reading

Bancroft, J.D. and Cook, H.C. (1984). Manual of histological techniques. Edinburgh. Churchill Livingstone.

Bancroft, J.D. and Stevens, A. (eds.) (1982). Theory and practice of histological techniques, 2nd Edn. Edinburgh. Churchill Livingstone.

Filipe, M.I. and Lake, B.D. (eds.) (1983). Histochemistry in pathology. Edinburgh. Churchill Livingstone.

Polak, J.M. and Van Noorden, S. (eds.) (1983). Immunocytochemistry. Bristol. Wright PSG.

Smith, A. and Bruton, J. (1977). A Colour Atlas of Histological Staining Techniques. Wolfe Medical Publications.

Weakley, B.S. (1981). A beginner's handbook in biological transmission electron microscopy, 2nd Edn. Edinburgh. Churchill Livingstone.

Index